Cardiovascular and Thoracic Imaging:
Trends, Perspectives and Prospects

Cardiovascular and Thoracic Imaging: Trends, Perspectives and Prospects

Editor

Mickaël Ohana

MDPI • Basel • Beijing • Wuhan • Barcelona • Belgrade • Manchester • Tokyo • Cluj • Tianjin

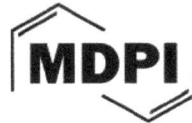

Editor
Mickaël Ohana
Strasbourg University Hospital
France

Editorial Office
MDPI
St. Alban-Anlage 66
4052 Basel, Switzerland

This is a reprint of articles from the Special Issue published online in the open access journal *Journal of Clinical Medicine* (ISSN 2077-0383) (available at: https://www.mdpi.com/journal/jcm/special_issues/Cardiovascular_Thoracic_Imaging_Perspectives_Prospects).

For citation purposes, cite each article independently as indicated on the article page online and as indicated below:

LastName, A.A.; LastName, B.B.; LastName, C.C. Article Title. *Journal Name* **Year**, *Volume Number*, Page Range.

ISBN 978-3-0365-3371-1 (Hbk)
ISBN 978-3-0365-3372-8 (PDF)

© 2022 by the authors. Articles in this book are Open Access and distributed under the Creative Commons Attribution (CC BY) license, which allows users to download, copy and build upon published articles, as long as the author and publisher are properly credited, which ensures maximum dissemination and a wider impact of our publications.

The book as a whole is distributed by MDPI under the terms and conditions of the Creative Commons license CC BY-NC-ND.

Contents

About the Editor vii

Trieu-Nghi Hoang-Thi, Guillaume Chassagnon, Thong Hua-Huy, Veronique Boussaud, Anh-Tuan Dinh-Xuan and Marie-Pierre Revel
Chronic Lung Allograft Dysfunction Post Lung Transplantation: A Review of Computed Tomography Quantitative Methods for Detection and Follow-Up
Reprinted from: *J. Clin. Med.* 2021, 10, 1608, doi:10.3390/jcm10081608 1

Salim Aymeric Si-Mohamed, Jade Miailhes, Pierre-Antoine Rodesch, Sara Boccalini, Hugo Lacombe, Valérie Leitman, Vincent Cottin, Loic Boussel and Philippe Douek
Spectral Photon-Counting CT Technology in Chest Imaging
Reprinted from: *J. Clin. Med.* 2021, 10, 5757, doi:10.3390/jcm10245757 13

Benjamin Longère, Julien Pagniez, Augustin Coisne, Hedi Farah, Michaela Schmidt, Christoph Forman, Valentina Silvestri, Arianna Simeone, Christos V Gkizas, Justin Hennicaux, Emma Cheasty, Solenn Toupin, David Montaigne and François Pontana
Right Ventricular Volume and Function Assessment in Congenital Heart Disease Using CMR Compressed-Sensing Real-Time Cine Imaging
Reprinted from: *J. Clin. Med.* 2021, 10, 1930, doi:10.3390/jcm10091930 31

Benjamin Longère, Christos V. Gkizas, Augustin Coisne, Lucas Grenier, Valentina Silvestri, Julien Pagniez, Arianna Simeone, Justin Hennicaux, Michaela Schmidt, Christoph Forman, Solenn Toupin, David Montaigne and François Pontana
60-S Retrogated Compressed Sensing 2D Cine of the Heart: Sharper Borders and Accurate Quantification
Reprinted from: *J. Clin. Med.* 2021, 10, 2417, doi:10.3390/jcm10112417 45

Cécile Chung, Sébastien Bommart, Sylvain Marchand-Adam, Mathieu Lederlin, Ludovic Fournel, Marie-Christine Charpentier, Lionel Groussin, Marie Wislez, Marie-Pierre Revel and Guillaume Chassagnon
Long-Term Imaging Follow-Up in DIPNECH: Multicenter Experience
Reprinted from: *J. Clin. Med.* 2021, 10, 2950, doi:10.3390/jcm10132950 61

François Laurent, Ilyes Benlala, Gael Dournes, Celine Gramond, Isabelle Thaon, Bénédicte Clin, Patrick Brochard, Antoine Gislard, Pascal Andujar, Soizick Chammings's, Justine Gallet, Aude Lacourt, Fleur Delva, Christophe Paris, Gilbert Ferretti and Jean-Claude Pairon
Interstitial Lung Abnormalities Detected by CT in Asbestos-Exposed Subjects Are More Likely Associated to Age
Reprinted from: *J. Clin. Med.* 2021, 10, 3130, doi:10.3390/jcm10143130 73

Benjamin Longère, Paul-Edouard Allard, Christos V Gkizas, Augustin Coisne, Justin Hennicaux, Arianna Simeone, Michaela Schmidt, Christoph Forman, Solenn Toupin, David Montaigne and François Pontana
Compressed Sensing Real-Time Cine Reduces CMR Arrhythmia-Related Artifacts
Reprinted from: *J. Clin. Med.* 2021, 10, 3274, doi:10.3390/jcm10153274 83

Anne-Claire Ortlieb, Aissam Labani, François Severac, Mi-Young Jeung, Catherine Roy and Mickaël Ohana
Impact of Morphotype on Image Quality and Diagnostic Performance of Ultra-Low-Dose Chest CT
Reprinted from: *J. Clin. Med.* 2021, 10, 3284, doi:10.3390/jcm10153284 97

Salim Aymeric Si-Mohamed, Lauria Marie Restier, Arthur Branchu, Sara Boccalini, Anaelle Congi, Arthur Ziegler, Danka Tomasevic, Thomas Bochaton, Loic Boussel and Philippe Charles Douek
Diagnostic Performance of Extracellular Volume Quantified by Dual-Layer Dual-Energy CT for Detection of Acute Myocarditis
Reprinted from: *J. Clin. Med.* **2021**, *10*, 3286, doi:10.3390/jcm10153286 . . . . **111**

About the Editor

Mickaël Ohana is a Professor of Radiology at Strasbourg University Hospital, specializing in cardiovascular and chest imaging. His main research interests are low-dose CT, coronary CTA, CT angiography, artificial intelligence and its applications to medical imaging.

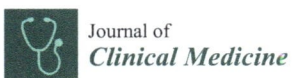

Review

Chronic Lung Allograft Dysfunction Post Lung Transplantation: A Review of Computed Tomography Quantitative Methods for Detection and Follow-Up

Trieu-Nghi Hoang-Thi [1,2,3], Guillaume Chassagnon [1], Thong Hua-Huy [3], Veronique Boussaud [4], Anh-Tuan Dinh-Xuan [3] and Marie-Pierre Revel [1,*]

1. AP-HP.Centre, Hôpital Cochin, Department of Radiology, Université de Paris, 75014 Paris, France htrieunghi@yahoo.fr (T.-N.H.-T.); guillaume.chassagnon@aphp.fr (G.C.)
2. Department of Diagnostic Imaging, Vinmec Central Park Hospital, Ho Chi Minh City 70000, Vietnam
3. AP-HP.Centre, Hôpital Cochin, Department of Respiratory Physiology, Université de Paris, 75014 Paris, France; huy-thong.hua@aphp.fr (T.H.-H.); anh-tuan.dinh-xuan.fr (A.-T.D.-X.)
4. AP-HP.Centre, Hôpital Cochin, Department of Pneumology, Université de Paris, 75014 Paris, France; veronique.boussaud@aphp.fr
* Correspondence: marie-pierre.revel@aphp.fr; Tel.: +33-1-5841-2471

Abstract: Chronic lung allograft dysfunction (CLAD) remains the leading cause of morbidity and mortality after lung transplantation. The term encompasses both obstructive and restrictive phenotypes, as well as mixed and undefined phenotypes. Imaging, in addition to pulmonary function tests, plays a major role in identifying the CLAD phenotype and is essential for follow-up after lung transplantation. Quantitative imaging allows for the performing of reader-independent precise evaluation of CT examinations. In this review article, we will discuss the role of quantitative imaging methods for evaluating the airways and the lung parenchyma on computed tomography (CT) images, for an early identification of CLAD and for prognostic estimation. We will also discuss their limits and the need for novel approaches to predict, understand, and identify CLAD in its early stages.

Keywords: lung transplantation; image processing; computer-assisted; pulmonary disease; chronic obstructive; bronchiolitis obliterans

Citation: Hoang-Thi, T.-N.; Chassagnon, G.; Hua-Huy, T.; Boussaud, V.; Dinh-Xuan, A.-T.; Revel, M.-P. Chronic Lung Allograft Dysfunction Post Lung Transplantation: A Review of Computed Tomography Quantitative Methods for Detection and Follow-Up. *J. Clin. Med.* **2021**, *10*, 1608. https://doi.org/10.3390/jcm10081608

Academic Editor: Takashi Ohtsuka

Received: 6 March 2021
Accepted: 8 April 2021
Published: 10 April 2021

Publisher's Note: MDPI stays neutral with regard to jurisdictional claims in published maps and institutional affiliations.

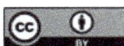

Copyright: © 2021 by the authors. Licensee MDPI, Basel, Switzerland. This article is an open access article distributed under the terms and conditions of the Creative Commons Attribution (CC BY) license (https://creativecommons.org/licenses/by/4.0/).

1. Introduction

Compared to other organ transplantation, lung transplantation remains associated with a poorer prognosis, with a median survival of only six years after transplantation [1]. The main cause of death beyond the first year is chronic lung allograft dysfunction (CLAD). This term refers to the deterioration of lung function as a result of chronic rejection and is not limited to an exclusively obstructive phenotype, referred to as bronchiolitis obstructive syndrome (BOS), but also includes a restrictive phenotype of chronic allograft dysfunction, termed restrictive allograft syndrome (RAS). The classification of CLAD phenotypes updated in 2019 by the International Society of Heart and Lung Transplantation (ISHLT) included BOS, accounting for 70% of allograft dysfunctions, and three other entities, RAS, mixed, and undefined phenotypes, representing the other 30% of phenotypes [2]. Their respective definitions are summarized in Table 1.

Hota et al. provided a comprehensive description of the different CLAD phenotypes on high-resolution CT [3]. RAS is associated with persistent parenchymal opacities and pleural thickening showing upper lung predominance, with pleuro parenchymal fibroelastosis on pathological examination, explaining the restrictive pattern [2,3]. Complementing pulmonary function tests (PFTs) with CT is thus mandatory not only to exclude other causes of lung function degradation but also to classify CLAD phenotypes. This classification is important for prognosis, with patients with a restrictive pattern of CLAD having worse survival [4]. Furthermore, Levy et al. [5] demonstrated that patients with undefined/unclassified CLAD phenotypes who had RAS-like opacities on chest imaging had significantly worse allograft survival than patients with the BOS phenotype. Suhling et al. [6] performed visual scoring of reticulations and consolidations in lung transplanted (LTx) patients and found poorer survival in patients with severe reticular changes. Imaging follow-up is especially important to detect CLAD in patients with single lung transplantation, because native lung disease may confound the interpretation of physiology [7].

Table 1. Definition of different CLAD phenotypes.

Phenotypes	Physiological Changes	Radiological Changes
CLAD (Chronic lung allograft dysfunction)	Persistent ≥ 20% decline in FEV1 (on the basis of 2 FEV1 values at least 3 weeks apart) compared with the baseline value, defined as the mean of the best 2 post-operative FEV1 measurement values, in the absence of other etiologies such as infection or acute rejection	
BOS (Bronchiolitis obliterans syndrome)	Persistent ≥ 20% decline in FEV1 compared with the baseline value (=CLAD definition) AND obstructive ventilatory defect (FEV1/forced vital capacity [FVC] < 0.7)	
RAS (Restrictive allograft syndrome)	Persistent ≥ 20% decline in FEV1 compared with the baseline value (=CLAD definition) AND ≥10% decline in TLC relative to baseline	Persistent opacities on chest imaging
Mixed phenotype	Persistent ≥ 20% decline in FEV1 compared with the baseline value (=CLAD definition) AND combination of obstructive and restrictive ventilatory defect (FEV1/FVC < 0.7 and a TLC ≤ 90% of baseline)	Persistent opacities on chest imaging
Undefined phenotype (1)	Persistent ≥ 20% decline in FEV1 compared with the baseline value (=CLAD definition) AND combination of obstructive and restrictive ventilatory defect (FEV1/FVC < 0.7 and a TLC ≤ 90% of baseline)	
Undefined phenotype (2)	Persistent ≥ 20% decline in FEV1 compared with the baseline value (=CLAD definition) AND obstructive ventilatory defect (FEV1/FVC < 0.7) and no decline in TLC	Persistent opacities on chest imaging

A switch from visual descriptive evaluation to quantitative automatic measurements has recently emerged in the field of medical imaging. Quantitative imaging has been mainly used for the evaluation of BOS, the obstructive phenotype of CLAD. The implementation of such imaging analysis tools for CLAD evaluation in LTx patients either directly confirms airway thickening and vascular remodeling in the allograft lung [8,9] or indirectly suggests their occurrence through air-trapping quantification [10,11]. Applying machine learning to imaging data analysis may further improve the management of CLAD [12]. In this review article, we will provide an overview of the CT quantification methods used to investigate CLAD of various phenotypes (see Figure 1 and Table 2), and discuss novel approaches to identify CLAD in its early stage. As sub-clinical chronic rejection compromises allograft integrity, there is a need to develop physiological and imaging tests allowing early detection of CLAD, with a potential role for quantitative imaging to serve as a biomarker, allowing early identification of CLAD [13].

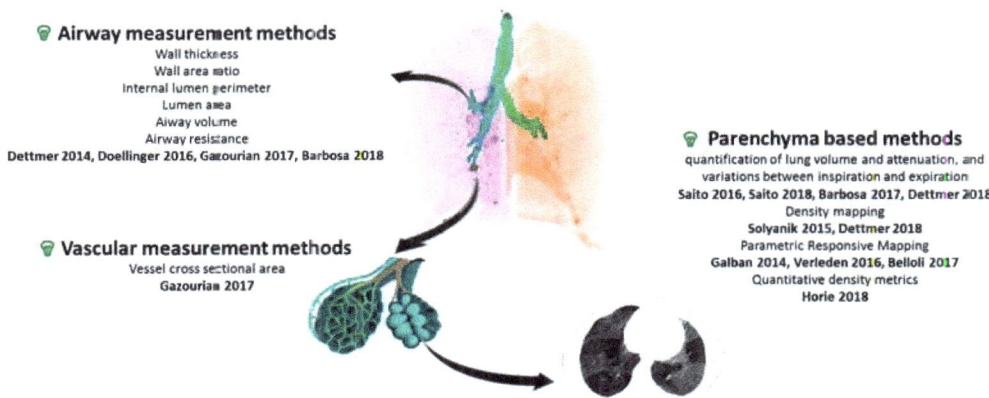

Figure 1. Overview of CT quantification methods for CLAD. CT: computer tomography, CLAD: chronic lung allograft dysfunction. Airway measurement methods [8,9,12,14], Vascular measurement methods [14], Parenchyma based methods [10,11,15–21].

Table 2. Overview of CT quantification methods for CLAD.

Author Year	Year	Study Design/Number of Patients	Time of CT Evaluation	Software	Main Quantification Parameters	Main Results
					Airway measurement methods	
Dettmer [9]	2014	Prospective study 141 patients (25 BOS+)	6, 12, 24 months after LTx	MeVis Airway Examiner	WT, WA%, WTdiff between inspiration and expiration on two selected bronchi B01 and B10	Greater WA% on inspiration in BOS+
Doellinger [8]	2016	Retrospective study 26 patients (12 BOS+)	All available CT scans after LTx	YACTA module v.1.0.7.16	ΔWT and ΔWA%: temporal change of WT and WA%;	Temporal changes of WT and WA% showed significant differences between BOS+ and BOS−
Gazourian [14]	2017	Retrospective study 66 patients (20 controls, 22 BOS non progressors and 24 BOS progressors)	non-volumetric CT closest to baseline FEV_1 and 2 follow-up CT scans	Airway Inspector (www.airwayinspector.org)	Internal lumen perimeter Lumen airway Airway vessel (A/V) ratio	Increase in the A/V ratio on follow-up CT scans for BOS progressors
Barbosa [12]	2018	Retrospective study 71 patients (41 BOS+)	2 CT scans (>3 months apart)	Mimics, TGrid 14.0 and Fluent 14.0	Airway volumes Airway resistances	Increase in central airway volume on expiratory CT in BOS+ Smaller airway volumes and airway surfaces and higher airway resistances at baseline in BOS developers
					Vascular measurement method	
Gazourian [14]	2017	Retrospective study 22 patients (13 BOS+)	2 volumetric CT angiographies after LTx	Bronchi: Airway Inspector Vessels: Upper thresholding (cut-off level of −500 HU) and use of a connected components technique	Vessel cross sectional area (CSA) Airway lumen area Airway/Vascular ratio (A/V ratio)	Overtime decrease in CSA in BOS+ Overtime Increase in A/V ratio in BOS+
					Parenchyma-based methods: quantification of air trapping	
Belloli [11]	2017	Retrospective study (22 BOS+ and controls matched by time from LTx; 52 BOS+)	Date of BOS	Lung segmentation: In-house algorithm Insp/Expiratory registration algorithm: Elastix	Parametric response mapping (PRM): Density-based quantification of air trapping (PRM^{fSAD}) and parenchymal disease (PRM^{PD})	FEV_1 decline associated with higher PRM^{fSAD} FEV_1 and FVC decline associated with higher PRM^{PD} $PRM^{fSAD} \geq 30\%$ strongest predictor of death

Table 2. Cont.

Author Year	Year	Study Design/Number of Patients	Time of CT Evaluation	Software	Main Quantification Parameters	Main Results
Verleden [10]	2016	Retrospective study 40 patients (20 BOS+)	CT scans before, at the time of and after of the diagnostic of BOS	Lung segmentation: In-house algorithm Insp/Expiratory registration algorithm: Elastix	Density-based quantification of air trapping (PRM^{fSAD}), parenchymal disease (PRM^{PD}), and normal lung (PRM^{Normal})	Increase in PRM^{fSAD} and decrease in PRM^{Normal} in BOS+ No difference in PRM^{fSAD} between BOS- and BOS+ before the diagnosis of BOS
Solyanik [15]	2015	Prospective study 147 patients (34 with air-trapping)	CT at 6 months after LTx	Not mentioned	Density based quantification of air trapping (EXP$_{-790 HU}$ to $_{-950 HU}$; E/I-MLD) Density mapping: voxel-to-voxel insp/expiration mapping	DM has the highest correlation to RV/TLC (r = 0.663, $p < 0.001$) DM and E/I-ratio MLD showed better correlation with RV/TLC than EXP$_{-790HU}$ to $_{-950HU}$
Barbosa [16]	2017	Retrospective study 174 patients (98 BOS+)	CTs within 9 years after LTx	ANTs package	- Lung volume in inspiration and expiration - Lung volume difference between insp and expiration - Density-based quantification of air trapping (EXP$_{<-856 HU}$, voxel volume with <75 HU increase on expiration)	Only 59% of qCT parameters associated with BOS+ BOS prediction model combining qCT and PFT parameters outperforms model based on PFTs alone in the unilateral LTx group
Dettmer [17]	2018	Prospective study 51 patients (17 BOS+)	Last CT within 1 year before BOS diagnostic First CT within 1 year after BOS diagnostic	Mevis Pulmo	Density based quantification of air trapping (E/I-MLD ratio, E/I Volumes, density percentiles)	Significant increase in E/I-Volumes and decrease in E/I-MLD in BOS+ Changes more pronounced in the lower lobes Highest AUC for 10th percentile on expiration (0.903) and E/I-MLD ratio (AUC: 0.886)
Horie [18]	2018	Retrospective study 74 patients (23 RAS, 51 BOS)	CT performed ±4 months from CLAD and/or RAS/BOS onset.	Lung segmentation on Vitrea workstation	Lung volume and MLD on inspiration Quantitative density metrics (QDM) defined as ratios of the right and left quantile weights of the density histogram on inspiratory CT	Significant difference of Lung volume and MLD in BOS and RAS patients Hazard ratio for death 3.2 times higher at the 75th percentile of QDM1 compared to the 25th percentile

Table 2. *Cont.*

Author Year	Year	Study Design/Number of Patients	Time of CT Evaluation	Software	Main Quantification Parameters	Main Results
Saito [20]	2016	Retrospective study 63 patients (19 RAS, 44 BOS)	CT performed at baseline and time of CLAD onset	Lung segmentation on Vitrea workstation	Lung volume on inspiration	Decrease in CT lung volume in RAS patients. CT volumetry < 90% baseline had an accuracy of 0.937 for differentiating RAS from BOS
Saito [21]	2018	Retrospective study 58 patients, 14 CLAD	CT performed 3, 6, and 12 months after LTx and once yearly thereafter	Lung segmentation on Synapse Vincent workstation	Lung volume on inspiration and expiration. Evaluation of Δlung volume over time (difference between inspiration and expiration)	Δlung volume onset/baseline significantly decreased in the CLAD group. 0.80 cutoff had an AUC of 0.87

LTx: lung transplantation; WT: wall thickness; WA%: wall area percentage = ratio bronchial wall/total area (bronchial wall+ bronchial lumen); WTdiff: difference of wall thickness between expiration and inspiration; A/V ratio: airway vessel ratio; ΔWT and ΔWA%: temporal changes of WT and WA%; PRM^{fSAD}: Parametric Response Mapping representing functional small airways disease; PRM^{PD}: Parametric Response Mapping representing parenchymal disease; PRM^{Normal}: Parametric Response Mapping representing normal pulmonary parenchyma; EXP$_{-790\ HU\ to\ -950\ HU}$: percentage of voxels with attenuation values from -790 HU to -950 HU on expiration; DM: density mapping; E/I-MLD: expiratory-to-inspiratory mean lung density ratio; E/I-Volumes: expiratory-to-inspiratory volume ratio; RV/TLC: residual volume/total lung capacity qCT: quantitative CT.

2. Airway Measurement Methods: Computer-Assisted Airway Morphometry

Since the most common phenotype of CLAD is that of BOS, quantitative methods allowing the direct assessment of the airways have been developed. BOS primarily affects the small airways, with diameters of less than 2 mm. Due to the limited spatial resolution of clinical CT scanners, new measurement methods had to be developed to allow the measurement of the density and wall thickness of the small airways [22]. Such a method made it possible to obtain values of the wall thickness of the small airways correlated with FEV1 in COPD patients [23]. Several software now available commercially make it possible to obtain an automatic segmentation of the bronchial tree and sections strictly perpendicular to the bronchial axis considered at different levels, as well as an automatic measurement of the bronchial wall thickness (WT) and the wall area ratio (WA%), the ratio of the airway wall area to the whole airway area.

Using the YACTA software [24], Doellinger et al. retrospectively examined a total of 2190 airway cross sections on CT scans performed within 11 years of follow-up of 26 LTx patients with at least one measurement in every lobe of the transplanted lung [8]. They showed significant differences between patients with and without BOS in term of changes over time of WA% and WT and concluded that bronchial wall thickening and luminal dilatation observed in lung transplant allograft rejection can be detected and quantified using computer-assisted airway morphometry. Gazourian et al., in a retrospective analysis of 22 patients, observed and increase in the air airway internal lumen perimeter (PI), and airway lumen area (AI) in the 13 patients developing BOS [14]. They used Airway Inspector (now renamed Chest Imaging Platform) for evaluating the third and fourth generation B1 and B10 airways. They also evaluated the pulmonary vessels cross-sectional areas (CSA) after upper thresholding (cut-off level of −500 HU) and use of a connected components technique on volumetric CT pulmonary angiogram to isolate the vessel cross sections. These authors also measured the airway/vessel ratios (A/V ratio) on non-volumetric CT scans. They found a statistically significant decrease in the vessel CSA in BOS patients and a significant increase in the airway/vessel ratio in BOS progressors. This observation is in line with known physiology, namely vasoconstriction in poorly ventilated areas due to small airways disease. These two studies (Doellinger [8] and Gazourian [14]), although both based on a limited number, showed differences between BOS and controls, but automated quantification of airway dimension was limited by the need for manual adjustments. In addition, the methods used do not translate into early identification or prognostic tools for CLAD.

Dettmer [9] evaluated 25 patients with BOS and 116 controls using MeVis Airway Examiner. WA% on inspiration was significantly greater in patients with BOS, but the variability of bronchial wall measurements was high and the values for the WA% on inspiration in patients with and without BOS overlapped considerably, due to variable underlying lung volumes. Even though this limitation could be overcome by performing spirometry-controlled CT acquisitions, the authors concluded to a limited value of WA% for establishing a diagnosis of BOS in individual patients.

Barbosa et al. [12] conducted a retrospective analysis of LTx patients who had paired inspiratory and expiratory CTs, with an objective to detect BOS 0-p stage, as indicator of early disease ($\geq$10% decline in FEV1 or $\geq$25% decline in forced expiratory flow 25–75%). Baseline prediction of BOS was performed in a cohort of 41 patients, of which 15 developed BOS. They measured the airway volumes and airway resistances after 3D analysis of the airways and lung lobes using three different commercially available software, Mimics, TGrid 14.0 and Fluent 14.0, for computational fluid dynamics simulations. The authors found that BOS patients experienced an increase in central airway volume on expiratory CT, whereas patients with other cause of FEV1 decline had a decrease in the central airway volume on inspiratory CT. According to the authors, these findings reflected an increase in the extent of air trapping and peribronchiolar fibrosis which characterizes the BOS phenotype of CLAD. Image post-processing included segmentation of the tracheobronchial tree down to the level of airways with a diameter of 1–2 mm which required manual correction and took 2 to 6 h per scan, which is the main limitation to consider the clinical use of this approach.

3. Lung Parenchyma Methods: Assessment of Lung Volume and Attenuation, and Their Variations between Inspiration and Expiration

Barbosa et al. [16], using the Advanced Normalization Tools (ANTs) software package, calculated the aerated lung volume in inspiration and expiration via exclusion of any voxel > −50 HU and then evaluated the volume change between inspiration and expiration as the difference between these two values, in a retrospective patient cohort excluding the RAS phenotype. In addition to volume change, two other quantitative parameters reflecting air trapping were evaluated: the volume of voxels with attenuation < −856 HU on expiration and the volume of voxels with an increase in attenuation <75 HU from inspiration to expiration following non-rigid registration between the inspiratory and expiratory imaging datasets. Only 59% of quantitative CT metrics were significantly correlated with BOS status in this study including 176 LTx patients, and none of the variables alone was a good predictor of BOS. However, a support vector machine (SVM) model based on the quantitative CT variables outperformed models using visual scoring of CT anomalies or PFT for BOS prediction after unilateral LTx.

Dettmer et al. [17] conducted a prospective evaluation with the objective to detect the BOS phenotype of CLAD in a cohort of 122 LTx patients. They performed CT acquisition with a spirometry-controlled technique at full inspiration and end of expiration and used Mevis Pulmo software, allowing volume measurement and histogram analysis (mean lung density/MLD, peak, percentiles) for the whole lung and separately for each lobe. They demonstrated that in patients with early-stage BOS, the lower lobe volume increased and the MLD decreased between the baseline and follow-up examinations, whereas the volume and MLD in the upper lobes remained nearly constant. The histogram parameters showing the highest accuracies for early BOS detection were the 10th percentile on expiration (AUC: 0.903) and the expiratory-to-inspiratory (E/I) MLD ratio (AUC: 0.886).

E/I MLD ratio is one of the multiple quantitative parameters used to evaluate the volume of air trapping in BOS. Solyanik et al. [15] evaluated two other automated methods to quantify air trapping, which had only slight differences with those previously mentioned in the study by Barbosa [16]: the lung volume having attenuation values ranging from −950 to −790 HU on expiratory CT scans (attenuation < −856 HU for Barbosa) and the lung volume with less than 80 HU change (<75 HU change for Barbosa) between inspiration and expiration. The latter requires non-rigid registration of inspiration-expiration CT-data and voxel-to-voxel mapping, which Solyanik described as "density mapping". Among the three evaluated methods, density mapping showed the best correlation with the ratio of residual volume to total lung capacity (RV/TLC).

Parametric response mapping, similar to density mapping, involves assessing the attenuation of each voxel on inspiration and expiration after applying an elastic registration algorithm. Voxels with attenuation ≥950 HU and < −810 HU at inspiration and < −856 at expiration are considered to represent functional small airways disease (PRMfSAD). Belloli et al. [11] evaluating a retrospective cohort of 52 LTx patients reported that PRMfSAD values ≥ 30% were the strongest predictor of survival in a multivariable model including BOS grade and baseline FEV1% predicted. Verleden et al. [10] used PRM to monitor BOS progression in a retrospective study including 20 BOS and 20 controls (no restrictive CLAD phenotype). They observed an increase at time of BOS diagnosis. They also reported that patients who died from BOS had significantly higher PRMfSAD than living patients. Galban et al. investigated the use of PRM as an imaging biomarker in the diagnosis of BOS. They found that PRMfSAD > 28% was highly indicative of BOS occurrence, whether a concurrent infection was present or not [19].

Other authors have developed quantitative methods only requiring inspiratory CT data. This was the case for Horie et al. [18], who evaluated CT lung density histograms on a single inspiratory CT in CLAD patients after lung segmentation. Indeed, lung fibrosis associated with the RAS phenotype of CLAD is likely to increase lung density, whereas mosaic perfusion secondary to BOS has an invert effect, both being detectable when analyzing the lung density histogram: the right-sided tail reflects processes increasing lung density whereas the left-sided tail reflects processes decreasing lung density, such as mosaic attenuation in areas of BOS. Their objective was threefold, to evaluate prognosis after CLAD onset, distinguish between BOS and RAS phenotypes, and evaluate the prognosis within BOS and RAS patient groups separately. They evaluated the quantitative density metrics (QDM) defined as ratios of the right and left quantile weights of the histogram, reflecting the left vs. right asymmetry of the histogram. There was a statistically significant difference in QDMs between RAS and BOS patients. Higher QDM values were significantly associated with decreased survival. The authors concluded that this quantitative analysis of CT images was associated with survival after the onset of CLAD and was able to differentiate RAS and BOS phenotypes. QDM measurement has been used by the same authors [25] to predict the risk of subsequent CLAD in patients with CLAD-0p, defined as a drop in FEV1 to 81–90% of baseline. Higher QDM values were associated with a shorter time between CLAD-0p-CT and CLAD.

Fewer quantitative CT methods have been developed for the RAS phenotype of CLAD. Measurement of inspiratory and expiratory CT lung volumes can be easily performed and CT volumetry has been shown to differentiate RAS patients from BOS patients due to the strong positive correlation between inspiratory lung CT volumes and TLC [20]. Computed tomography is particularly useful for detecting CLAD affecting a single lung [7,21], because the unaffected contralateral lung compensates for the deficit in lung function on PFTs. A decrease over time in the difference between inspiratory and expiratory lung volumes has been reported for obstructive and restrictive CLAD phenotypes [21].

PRM is another method allowing quantitative evaluation of patients with the RAS phenotype of CLAD, who have persistent parenchymal opacities and pleural thickening. Voxels with attenuation values ≥ -810 HU at inspiration represent parenchymal disease (PRMPD). In the study by Belloli et al. [11] evaluating 22 LTx patients, those with concurrent declines in both FEV1 and FVC (e.g., RAS phenotype) were found to have significantly more PRMPD than their control group, even after adjusting for age, baseline FEV1% predicted, and baseline FVC % predicted. The prognostic value of PRMPD was not mentioned and should probably be evaluated in a larger patient group.

To be clinically useful, quantitative methods should not require multiple complex algorithms or manual steps to correct segmentation, which is the case with computer-assisted airway morphometry. In addition, these methods only assess the BOS phenotype of CLAD and have limited diagnostic value. Simpler methods based on CT volumetry are more accessible, with the assessment of lung volume and lobe attenuation on inspiration and expiration of interest for all CLAD phenotypes.

Regarding the processing of imaging data by artificial intelligence for CLAD diagnosis, the current literature is scarce. Classical machine learning methods such as the support vector machine (SVM) using quantitative CT metrics were of interest to diagnose BOS following unilateral LTx, as previously mentioned [16]. SVM was also used to evaluate multiple combinations of functional respiratory indexes (FRI) for BOS prediction at six months after transplantation [12]. A maximal accuracy of 85% was obtained by combining three baseline FRI features: the right middle lobe volume at total lung capacity (inspiratory CT scan), the right upper lobe airway resistance and the central airway surface at functional residual capacity (expiratory CT). Deep learning represents a major advance in the field of artificial intelligence applied to medical imaging, but requires a large amount of data [26,27]. As previously highlighted, most series on quantitative imaging for CLAD evaluation post LTx are based on a limited number of patients, because lung transplantation is not a common procedure. In 2015, only 14 centers reported performing 50 or more LTx per year [28]. Therefore, the standardization of imaging follow-up and data sharing through a common registry is crucial before considering the development of deep learning algorithms for the prediction and early diagnosis of CLAD.

4. Conclusions

Quantitative imaging methods offer the opportunity to perform reader-independent assessment of the airways and lung parenchyma in LTx patients. Although said to be automatic, most methods still require significant time-consuming manual corrections, and require the availability of segmentation and elastic registration algorithms, which limits their direct use in clinical routine. However, the results obtained in the studies published to date demonstrate the prognostic impact of methods such as parametric response mapping quantifying functional small airway disease (PRMfSAD) or quantitative density metrics (QDM). The performance for the prediction or early detection of CLAD needs to be strengthened, which could be an objective of deep learning-based methods. Developing prediction models is indeed important to improve outcomes for patients who are developing CLAD and better understand the underlining pathophysiology.

Author Contributions: Conceptualization, T.-N.H.-T. and M.-P.R.; methodology, G.C.; Literature research T.-N.H.-T. and T.H.-H.; writing—original draft preparation, T.-N.H.-T.; writing—review and editing, all authors.; supervision, M.-P.R. and A.-T.D.-X. All authors have read and agreed to the published version of the manuscript.

Funding: This review article received no external funding.

Informed Consent Statement: Not applicable.

Data Availability Statement: Not applicable.

Conflicts of Interest: The authors declare no conflict of interest.

References

1. Chambers, D.C.; Yusen, R.D.; Cherikh, W.S.; Goldfarb, S.B.; Kucheryavaya, A.Y.; Khusch, K.; Levvey, B.J.; Lund, L.H.; Meiser, B.; Rossano, J.W.; et al. The Registry of the International Society for Heart and Lung Transplantation: Thirty-Fourth Adult Lung and Heart-Lung Transplantation Report—2017; Focus Theme: Allograft Ischemic Time. *J. Heart Lung. Transplant.* **2017**, *36*, 1047–1059. [CrossRef]
2. Verleden, G.M.; Glanville, A.R.; Lease, E.D.; Fisher, A.J.; Calabrese, F.; Corris, P.A.; Ensor, C.R.; Gottlieb, J.; Hachem, R.R.; Lama, V.; et al. Chronic Lung Allograft Dysfunction: Definition, Diagnostic Criteria, and Approaches to Treatment—A Consensus Report from the Pulmonary Council of the ISHLT. *J. Heart Lung. Transplant.* **2019**, *38*, 493–503. [CrossRef]
3. Hota, P.; Dass, C.; Kumaran, M.; Simpson, S. High-Resolution CT Findings of Obstructive and Restrictive Phenotypes of Chronic Lung Allograft Dysfunction: More Than Just Bronchiolitis Obliterans Syndrome. *Am. J. Roentgenol.* **2018**, *211*, W13–W21. [CrossRef] [PubMed]
4. DerHovanessian, A.; Todd, J.L.; Zhang, A.; Li, N.; Mayalall, A.; Finlen Copeland, C.A.; Shino, M.; Pavlisko, E.N.; Wallace, W.D.; Gregson, A.; et al. Validation and Refinement of Chronic Lung Allograft Dysfunction Phenotypes in Bilateral and Single Lung Recipients. *Ann. Am. Thorac. Soc.* **2016**, *13*, 627–635. [CrossRef] [PubMed]
5. Levy, L.; Huszti, E.; Renaud-Picard, B.; Berra, G.; Kawashima, M.; Takahagi, A.; Fuchs, E.; Ghany, R.; Moshkelgosha, S.; Keshavjee, S.; et al. Risk Assessment of Chronic Lung Allograft Dysfunction Phenotypes: Validation and Proposed Refinement of the 2019 International Society for Heart and Lung Transplantation Classification System. *J. Heart Lung. Transplant.* **2020**, *39*, 761–770. [CrossRef]
6. Suhling, H.; Dettmer, S.; Greer, M.; Fuehner, T.; Avsar, M.; Haverich, A.; Welte, T.; Gottlieb, J. Phenotyping Chronic Lung Allograft Dysfunction Using Body Plethysmography and Computed Tomography. *Am. J. Transplant.* **2016**, *16*, 3163–3170. [CrossRef] [PubMed]
7. Philippot, Q.; Debray, M.-P.; Bun, R.; Frija-Masson, J.; Bunel, V.; Morer, L.; Roux, A.; Picard, C.; Jebrak, G.; Dauriat, G.; et al. Use of CT-SCAN Score and Volume Measures to Early Identify Restrictive Allograft Syndrome in Single Lung Transplant Recipients. *J. Heart Lung. Transplant.* **2020**, *39*, 125–133. [CrossRef]
8. Doellinger, F.; Weinheimer, O.; Zwiener, I.; Mayer, E.; Buhl, R.; Fahlenkamp, U.L.; Dueber, C.; Achenbach, T. Differences of Airway Dimensions between Patients with and without Bronchiolitis Obliterans Syndrome after Lung Transplantation-Computer-Assisted Quantification of Computed Tomography. *Eur. J. Radiol.* **2016**, *85*, 1414–1420. [CrossRef]
9. Dettmer, S.; Peters, L.; de Wall, C.; Schaefer-Prokop, C.; Schmidt, M.; Warnecke, G.; Gottlieb, J.; Wacker, F.; Shin, H. Bronchial Wall Measurements in Patients after Lung Transplantation: Evaluation of the Diagnostic Value for the Diagnosis of Bronchiolitis Obliterans Syndrome. *PLoS ONE* **2014**, *9*, e93783. [CrossRef]
10. Verleden, S.E.; Vos, R.; Vandermeulen, E.; Ruttens, D.; Bellon, H.; Heigl, T.; Van Raemdonck, D.E.; Verleden, G.M.; Lama, V.; Ross, B.D.; et al. Parametric Response Mapping of Bronchiolitis Obliterans Syndrome Progression after Lung Transplantation. *Am. J. Transplant.* **2016**, *16*, 3262–3269. [CrossRef]

11. Belloli, E.A.; Degtiar, I.; Wang, X.; Yanik, G.A.; Stuckey, L.J.; Verleden, S.E.; Kazerooni, E.A.; Ross, B.D.; Murray, S.; Galbán, C.J.; et al. Parametric Response Mapping as an Imaging Biomarker in Lung Transplant Recipients. *Am. J. Respir. Crit. Care Med.* **2017**, *195*, 942–952. [CrossRef]
12. Barbosa, E.J.M.; Lanclus, M.; Vos, W.; Van Holsbeke, C.; De Backer, W.; De Backer, J.; Lee, J. Machine Learning Algorithms Utilizing Quantitative CT Features May Predict Eventual Onset of Bronchiolitis Obliterans Syndrome After Lung Transplantation. *Acad. Radiol.* **2018**, *25*, 1201–1212. [CrossRef]
13. Tissot, A.; Danger, R.; Claustre, J.; Magnan, A.; Brouard, S. Early Identification of Chronic Lung Allograft Dysfunction: The Need of Biomarkers. *Front. Immunol.* **2019**, *10*, 1681. [CrossRef]
14. Gazourian, L.; Ash, S.; Meserve, E.E.K.; Diaz, A.; Estepar, R.S.J.; El-Chemaly, S.Y.; Rosas, I.O.; Divo, M.; Fuhlbrigge, A.L.; Camp, P.C.; et al. Quantitative Computed Tomography Assessment of Bronchiolitis Obliterans Syndrome after Lung Transplantation. *Clin. Transplant.* **2017**, *31*. [CrossRef] [PubMed]
15. Solyanik, O.; Hollmann, P.; Dettmer, S.; Kaireit, T.; Schaefer-Prokop, C.; Wacker, F.; Vogel-Claussen, J.; Shin, H. Quantification of Pathologic Air Trapping in Lung Transplant Patients Using CT Density Mapping: Comparison with Other CT Air Trapping Measures. *PLoS ONE* **2015**, *10*, e0139102. [CrossRef] [PubMed]
16. Barbosa, E.M.; Simpson, S.; Lee, J.C.; Tustison, N.; Gee, J.; Shou, H. Multivariate Modeling Using Quantitative CT Metrics May Improve Accuracy of Diagnosis of Bronchiolitis Obliterans Syndrome after Lung Transplantation. *Comput. Biol. Med.* **2017**, *89*, 275–281. [CrossRef] [PubMed]
17. Dettmer, S.; Suhling, H.; Klingenberg, I.; Otten, O.; Kaireit, T.; Fuge, J.; Kuhnigk, J.M.; Gottlieb, J.; Haverich, A.; Welte, T.; et al. Lobe-Wise Assessment of Lung Volume and Density Distribution in Lung Transplant Patients and Value for Early Detection of Bronchiolitis Obliterans Syndrome. *Eur. J. Radiol.* **2018**, *106*, 137–144. [CrossRef] [PubMed]
18. Horie, M.; Salazar, P.; Saito, T.; Binnie, M.; Brock, K.; Yasufuku, K.; Azad, S.; Keshavjee, S.; Martinu, T.; Paul, N. Quantitative Chest CT for Subtyping Chronic Lung Allograft Dysfunction and Its Association with Survival. *Clin. Transplant.* **2018**, *32*, e13233. [CrossRef] [PubMed]
19. Galbán, C.J.; Boes, J.L.; Bule, M.; Kitko, C.L.; Couriel, D.R.; Johnson, T.D.; Lama, V.; Telenga, E.D.; van den Berge, M.; Rehemtulla, A.; et al. Parametric Response Mapping as an Indicator of Bronchiolitis Obliterans Syndrome after Hematopoietic Stem Cell Transplantation. *Biol. Blood Marrow Transplant.* **2014**, *20*, 1592–1598. [CrossRef] [PubMed]
20. Saito, T.; Horie, M.; Sato, M.; Nakajima, D.; Shoushtarizadeh, H.; Binnie, M.; Azad, S.; Hwang, D.M.; Machuca, T.N.; Waddell, T.K.; et al. Low-Dose Computed Tomography Volumetry for Subtyping Chronic Lung Allograft Dysfunction. *J. Heart Lung. Transplant.* **2016**, *35*, 59–66. [CrossRef]
21. Saito, M.; Chen-Yoshikawa, T.F.; Nakamoto, Y.; Kayawake, H.; Tokuno, J.; Ueda, S.; Yamagishi, H.; Gochi, F.; Okabe, R.; Takahagi, A.; et al. Unilateral Chronic Lung Allograft Dysfunction Assessed by Biphasic Computed Tomographic Volumetry in Bilateral Living-Donor Lobar Lung Transplantation. *Transplant. Direct* **2018**, *4*, e398. [CrossRef] [PubMed]
22. Weinheimer, O.; Achenbach, T.; Bletz, C.; Duber, C.; Kauczor, H.U.; Heussel, C.P. About Objective 3-d Analysis of Airway Geometry in Computerized Tomography. *IEEE Trans. Med. Imaging* **2008**, *27*, 64–74. [CrossRef]
23. Achenbach, T.; Weinheimer, O.; Biedermann, A.; Schmitt, S.; Freudenstein, D.; Goutham, E.; Kunz, R.P.; Buhl, R.; Dueber, C.; Heussel, C.P. MDCT Assessment of Airway Wall Thickness in COPD Patients Using a New Method: Correlations with Pulmonary Function Tests. *Eur. Radiol.* **2008**, *18*, 2731–2738. [CrossRef] [PubMed]
24. Achenbach, T.; Weinheimer, O.; Buschsieweke, C.; Heussel, C.P.; Thelen, M.; Kauczor, H.U. Fully automatic detection and quantification of emphysema on thin section MD-CT of the chest by a new and dedicated software. *Rofo* **2004**, *176*, 1409–1415. [CrossRef] [PubMed]
25. Horie, M.; Levy, L.; Houbois, C.; Salazar, P.; Saito, T.; Pakkal, M.; O'Brien, C.; Sajja, S.; Brock, K.; Yasufuku, K.; et al. Lung Density Analysis Using Quantitative Chest CT for Early Prediction of Chronic Lung Allograft Dysfunction. *Transplantation* **2019**, *103*, 2645–2653. [CrossRef] [PubMed]
26. Chassagnon, G.; Vakalopoulou, M.; Paragios, N.; Revel, M.-P. Artificial Intelligence Applications for Thoracic Imaging. *Eur. J. Radiol.* **2020**, *123*, 108774. [CrossRef] [PubMed]
27. Chassagnon, G.; Vakalopoulou, M.; Paragios, N.; Revel, M.-P. Deep Learning: Definition and Perspectives for Thoracic Imaging. *Eur. Radiol.* **2020**, *30*, 2021–2030. [CrossRef]
28. Chambers, D.C.; Cherikh, W.S.; Harhay, M.O.; Hayes, D.; Hsich, E.; Khush, K.K.; Meiser, B.; Potena, L.; Rossano, J.W.; Toll, A.E.; et al. The International Thoracic Organ Transplant Registry of the International Society for Heart and Lung Transplantation: Thirty-Sixth Adult Lung and Heart-Lung Transplantation Report-2019; Focus Theme: Donor and Recipient Size Match. *J. Heart Lung. Transplant.* **2019**, *38*, 1042–1055. [CrossRef]

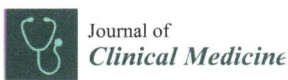

Review

Spectral Photon-Counting CT Technology in Chest Imaging

Salim Aymeric Si-Mohamed [1,2,*], Jade Miailhes [2], Pierre-Antoine Rodesch [1], Sara Boccalini [1,2], Hugo Lacombe [1], Valérie Leitman [1], Vincent Cottin [3], Loïc Boussel [1,2] and Philippe Douek [1,2]

[1] INSA-Lyon, University of Lyon, University Claude-Bernard Lyon 1, UJM-Saint-Étienne, CNRS Inserm, CREATIS UMR 5220, U1206, 69621 Lyon, France; rodesch@creatis.insa-lyon.fr (P.-A.R.); sara.boccalini@chu-lyon.fr (S.B.); Hugo.Lacombe1@phelma.grenoble-inp.fr (H.L.); vleitman77@gmail.com (V.L.); loic.boussel@chu-lyon.fr (L.B.); philippe.douek@chu-lyon.fr (P.D.)
[2] Radiology Department, Hospices Civils de Lyon, 69500 Lyon, France; jade.miailhes@gmail.com
[3] National Reference Center for Rare Pulmonary Diseases, Louis Pradel Hospital, Hospices Civils de Lyon, UMR 754, INRAE, Claude Bernard University Lyon 1, Member of ERN-LUNG, 69677 Lyon, France; vincent.cottin@chu-lyon.fr
* Correspondence: salim.si-mohamed@chu-lyon.fr; Tel.: +33-04-7235-73-35; Fax: +33-04-7235-72-91

Abstract: The X-ray imaging field is currently undergoing a period of rapid technological innovation in diagnostic imaging equipment. An important recent development is the advent of new X-ray detectors, i.e., photon-counting detectors (PCD), which have been introduced in recent clinical prototype systems, called PCD computed tomography (PCD-CT) or photon-counting CT (PCCT) or spectral photon-counting CT (SPCCT) systems. PCD allows a pixel up to 200 microns pixels at iso-center, which is much smaller than that can be obtained with conventional energy integrating detectors (EID). PCDs have also a higher dose efficiency than EID mainly because of electronic noise suppression. In addition, the energy-resolving capabilities of these detectors allow generating spectral basis imaging, such as the mono-energetic images or the water/iodine material images as well as the K-edge imaging of a contrast agent based on atoms of high atomic number. In recent years, studies have therefore been conducted to determine the potential of PCD-CT as an alternative to conventional CT for chest imaging.

Keywords: thorax; lung; diagnostic imaging; computed tomography; photon-counting detectors

1. Introduction

Chest imaging is constantly evolving, and the demand for diagnostic performance is growing in many areas, such as lung cancer, detection of pulmonary nodules, chronic obstructive pulmonary disease, as well as evaluation and follow-up of interstitial lung diseases (ILD). While CT is the most powerful tool currently available for this purpose, it has many limitations such that accurate diagnosis often requires additional histological analyses or other non-radiological examinations.

Photon-counting detector computed tomography (PCD-CT) technology is a new CT modality that has gained increasing interest in all areas of imaging, including musculoskeletal, digestive, cardiovascular, pulmonary, and molecular imaging [1–6]. Contrary to energy integrated detectors (EID) found in current standard CT scanners, PCD are made of compounds, such as silicon, cadmium-telluride, or cadmium-zinc-telluride, to directly convert each X-ray photon into an electric pulse, allowing resolution of the energy of the photons. This characteristic allows better intrinsic technical performance by reducing noise, increasing spatial resolution, decreasing beam hardening, and decreasing X-ray doses [7,8]. In addition, the energy-resolving capabilities of these detectors allow to generate spectral basis images, such as the monoenergetic images or water/iodine material images as well as the K-edge images of a contrast agent based on atoms of high atomic number. Taken together, PCD-CT provides new diagnostic perspectives compared to the conventional EID found in current CT systems. Studies have therefore been conducted in recent years, mainly limited to non-contrast lung imaging, to determine the potential of PCD-CT as an alternative to conventional CT. In the present review, we will discuss these studies and explore the perspectives of PCD-CT for chest imaging.

2. Technical Aspects
2.1. Photon-Counting Detector Technology

PCD are a recently developed technology seen as the future of X-ray measurement; the design of these detectors differs from that of EID, which are commonly used in clinical practice (Figure 1). The EID use a scintillator material transforming the incoming X-ray into visible light that is then captured by a photo-diode. The deposited energy in the pixel is integrated by an application-specific integrated circuit (ASIC) that produces a current proportional to the energy of the incoming photon. In contrast, the PCD are made of a semi-conductor material that directly converts the incoming photon to electrical charges, which migrate into a counting ASIC (Figure 1). This process is called direct conversion (by opposition to indirect conversion). The ASIC shapes a voltage pulse proportional to the incoming photon energy. From the amplitude of the pulse the PCD can differentiate photons according to their energy (Figure 2). PCD-CT can operate in two different modes: conventional or spectral. In the conventional mode, photons are not discriminated according to their energy but are only summed; "conventional images" are those computed from the attenuation of all counted photons. This corresponds to the single energy CT (SECT). The direct conversion design fundamentally improves three major aspects of X-ray SECT imaging: the size of the detector pixel, the reduction of the electronic noise, and the energy weighting in the analogical output signal. The resulting benefits of these aspects are detailed in the next section.

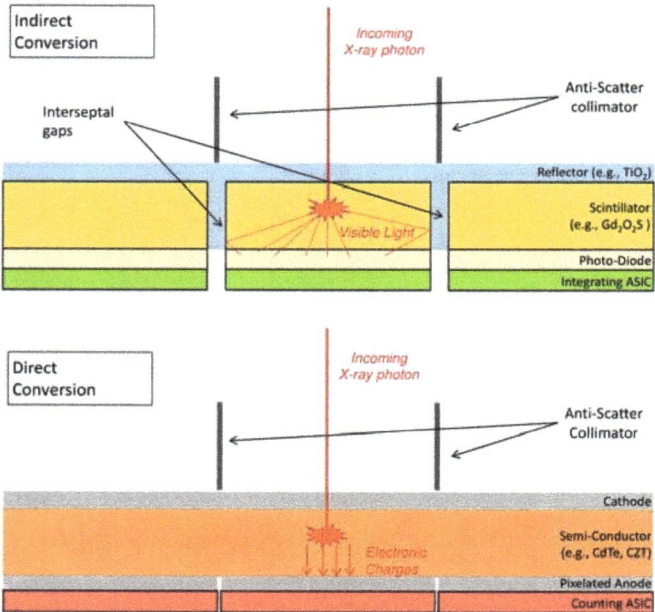

Figure 1. Schematic representation of photon detection technologies: energy-integrating (**top**) and photon-counting detectors (**bottom**).

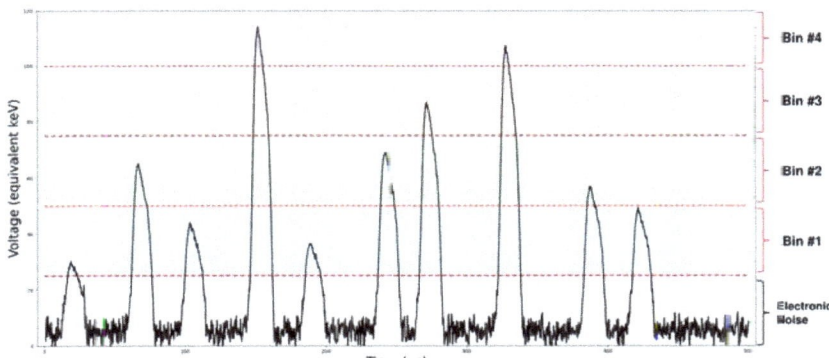

Figure 2. Example of a 500 ns signal output of a photon-counting detector pixel.

2.2. Benefits for Conventional Images

2.2.1. Spatial Resolution

Because the scintillator can produce visible photons in each direction, the EID pixels require separation by a reflector material (Figure 1). This leads to an interseptal gap between pixels that critically decreases the ratio of effective sensitive area to detector area when the pixel size becomes too small. The subsequent major loss of efficiency with respect to exposure limits the size of EID to 0.5 mm at iso-center in normal resolution for most of the current clinical system. PCD pixel pitch is not technically limited and can reach 0.19–0.225 mm at the iso-center in the latest full-body prototypes [9–12].

The most recent ultra-high-resolution (UHR) EID-CT uses EID made by a different manufacturing process than conventional ones [13]; the septa gap is thinner and closer to the thickness of the anti-scatter collimators (Figure 1). This leads to 0.25-mm voxel element at iso-center, which fills the gap between standard EID and PCD in terms of reconstructed voxel size for lung imaging [14]. However, some methods have shown promising results to correct scatter without a pre-detector collimator [15], even for PCD [16]. This anti-scatter grid removal would increase the sensitive area of PCD and not EID. Moreover, interseptal gaps prohibit the possibility for subpixel resolution, which is a process that better estimates the photon reaching point for a pixel based on the adjacent pixels [17].

To the best of our knowledge, a comparison of the dose efficiency between EID and PCD for a large detector panel with 0.25-mm voxel element size is not yet available. Even with the same this geometry configuration, the PCD still benefit from technical advantages described in the next subsections.

2.2.2. Reduction of Electronic Noise

According to the number of available thresholds (between 3 and 8 according to PCD manufacturer), several measurement bins can be defined (Figure 2) [9,11,12]. The first threshold is set just above the electronic noise level and suppresses it from the final counts, which cannot be done for EIDs, and therefore, electronic noise is added to the integrated energy. This means the noise in the reconstructed image is lower with PCD than with EID for the same dose.

2.2.3. Contrast Improvement

In addition to noise reduction, another aspect improving contrast-to-noise ratio (CNR) is the energy weighting of each incoming photon. As the linear attenuation coefficient decreases with energy, lower energy provides greater contrast, for example, when differentiating water from calcium [18] (Figure 3). Whereas EID produce a signal proportional to the incoming energy for one photon (linear weight), PCD will generate only one count irrespective of the photon measured (constant weight).

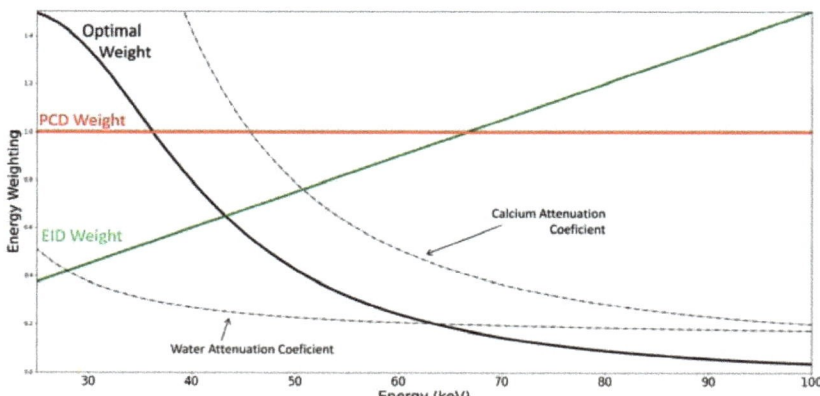

Figure 3. Energy weighting of energy integrating detectors (EID) and photon-counting detectors (PCD). The optimal weight for differentiating calcium from water is derived from the attenuation coefficients subtraction (dashed lines).

2.2.4. Reduction of Beam Hardening

The constant weight also reduces beam hardening artifacts in conventional images. Beam hardening is due to a difference in mean energies between the incident and the attenuated spectra, and the proportional weighting of EID increases this difference, which is not the case for the constant weighting of PCD [8,19].

2.2.5. Dose Efficiency

The advantages described above of PCD over EID lead to a better dose efficiency, as demonstrated by several studies [9,20–23]. The effect of this dose efficiency can be either to produce the same image quality for the same dose or to investigate new protocols. In addition, iterative reconstruction can decrease noise levels in reconstructed CT images. Combined with the emergence of iterative reconstruction, PCD-CT enables either the reconstruction with a larger matrix (1024 × 1024 or 2048 × 2048) or the efficiency of ultra-low dose protocols [9,22].

2.3. Spectral Mode

Recently, progress in informatics (high storage capacity, high-speed computation reconstruction) has allowed for spectral reconstructions in clinical practice through dual-energy CT (DECT) devices. However, DECT systems require major modification in their architecture compared to single energy CT [1]. While PCD-CT has the advantage to be able to run in both conventional and spectral mode, using a traditional X-ray source and CT geometry allows different types of images that are described in following subsections.

2.3.1. Virtual Monoenergetic (VMI) Images

PCD have the possibility to provide spectral measurement bins by differentiating incoming photons according to their energy (Figure 2). This spectral information can be used to reconstruct VMI [23]. VMIs are computed from spectral information at a (virtual) selected energy leading to beam hardening artifact reduction. Conversely, conventional images are the reconstruction of the attenuation coefficient averaged over the measured spectrum. VMIs can be reconstructed from either a PCD or a DECT acquisition. At low energies, VMIs allow a boost of the photoelectric effect such as the iodine boost in the presence of an iodinated contrast agent. This may allow a better depiction of the vessel lumen [24], while at high energies, VMI are robust to metal artifacts [25]. Another metal artifact-reduction technique is the reconstruction of an image using only photons measured over 70 keV. The resulting high-threshold image presents an increased CNR compared to conventional images in presence of metal artifacts [26].

2.3.2. K-edge Imaging

K-edge materials are a type of material with a discontinuity in their attenuation coefficient (Figure 4). This spectral singularity allows for an accurate contrast agent identification in the reconstructed volume [27]. Imaging of a K-edge material, known as K-edge imaging, requires the measurement of at least three energy bins, which is not feasible with DECT [1]. To be detected for clinical imaging, this effect must be within the energy range of the diagnostic X-ray that is between 40 and 140 keV. Unfortunately, iodine is not a good candidate because of the photon starvation around its K-edge, which is 33.3 keV. Hence, new contrast agents for CT should be designed and validated for K-edge imaging using high atomic-number atoms, such as gadolinium, gold, or bismuth (Figure 4).

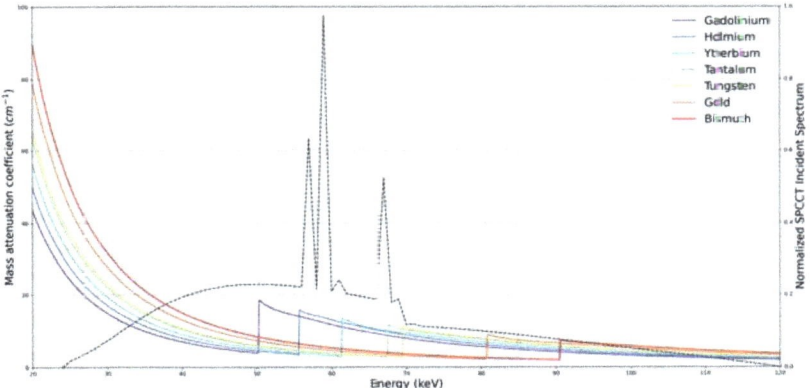

Figure 4. Attenuation coefficients of contrast agents with a K-edge in the medical energy range.

2.4. Conclusions

In this section detailing technical aspects, we introduced the three main advantages of PCD over EID for conventional imaging: smaller detector pixel, electronic noise reduction, and more efficient energy weighting of photons. These advantages have been demonstrated to improve conventional image quality in pre-clinical and preliminary clinical studies. However, this is not the only strong point of PCD-CT, as it can perform simultaneously spectral mode to study VMIs and K-edge contrast agents, which may open to new and promising applications.

3. Pre-Clinical and Clinical Applications

3.1. Parenchyma Imaging

Despite the recent availability of high-resolution CT (HRCT), evaluation of lung parenchyma integrity is a daily challenge for the radiologist. The principal reason is that radiological evaluation is sometimes limited by the fine semiology of the anatomical structures of the lung lobule [28]; pathological analysis therefore remains the technique of choice in case of diagnostic uncertainty [29]. However, due to its high spatial resolution, PCD-CT systems could revolutionize the evaluation of the lung. Accordingly, numerous studies have investigated PCD-CT imaging of the parenchyma by studying the influence of the reconstruction parameters, such as the matrix size, the slice thickness, and the iterative algorithms recently made available for this new technology.

For instance, Bartlett et al. [30] demonstrated in patients the value of using a 1024 matrix with a high-frequency filter (Q65) with a limited field-of-view (FOV) PCD-CT system, in comparison with a 512 and 1024 matrix and standard detailed filter (E46) with

PCD-CT and EID-CT. These reconstruction parameters were used to convey the high spatial resolution of the PCD-CT system, which improved the depiction of the lung parenchyma structures, such as the bronchi and morphological features of lesions (e.g., nodule, ground-glass nodules). Recently, on a different PCD-CT system [9], we demonstrated in human volunteer with a large FOV and a 1024 matrix, that lung structures, such as fissures, distal airways, and vessels, were of greater conspicuity and sharpness with better overall image quality than standard CT, despite a 23% flux reduction (Figure 5). Interestingly, the noise was also better rated by three experienced chest radiologists who noted a particular texture that characterizes high-frequency noise. In this study, we showed that the UHR parameters allowed to depict a 178-µm line width on a line pair phantom, which was enabled by a spatial resolution at 22.3 lp/cm at 10% modulation transfer function. Similarly, Leng et al. [10] reported in patients with a different PCD-CT system the value of an UHR mode for small lung structures using a sharp filter with a spatial frequency cutoff of 32.4 lp/cm, a 1024 matrix, and 0.25 slice thickness in comparison to a standard (macro) and sharp mode. The sharp and UHR modes showed similar modulation transfer functions, both better than for macro mode; 10% modulation transfer function value was 9.48 lp/cm for macro, 16.05 lp/cm for sharp, and 17.69 lp/cm for UHR modes.

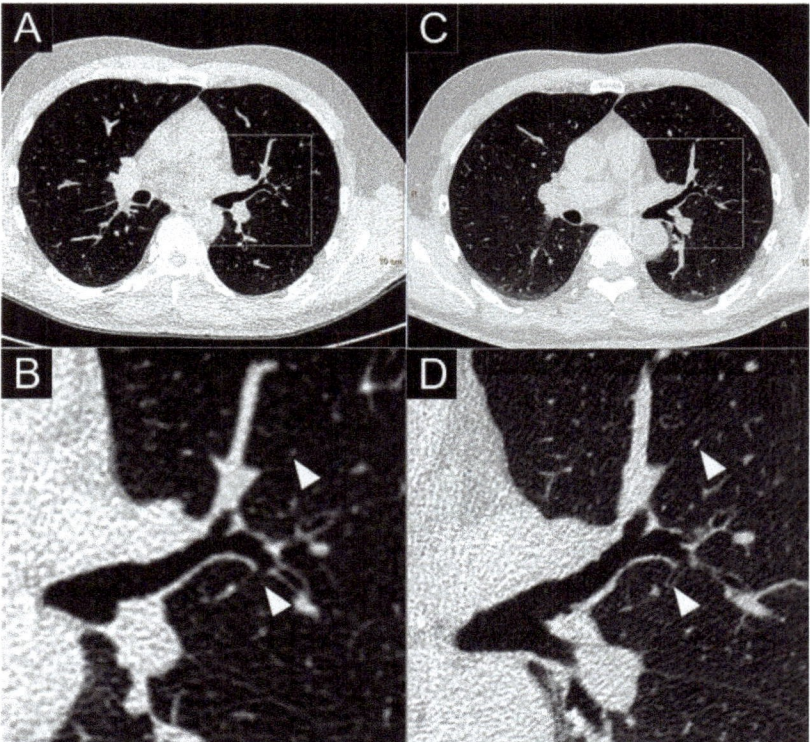

Figure 5. Comparison of high-resolution lung imaging between a conventional CT (Brilliance 64; Philips Haifa, Israel; (**A**,**B**)), a clinical prototype PCD-CT (SPCCT; Philips; (**C**,**D**)), and in a human volunteer. Close-up views on the left pulmonary hilum found a greater overall image quality as well as better depiction and a greater number of small structures (bronchial wall, vessels; white arrows).

Taken together, these studies show the potential for more accurate parenchyma evaluation in vitro as well as in human volunteers and patients with the UHR mode of the PCD-CT technology that requires confirmation in a prospective clinical study.

3.2. Nodule Imaging

Lung nodule imaging is a challenging task that necessitates an accurate characterization of the morphological features of a nodule [31]. In recent years, several studies have proven the performance of PCD-CT in the detection and morphological characterization of pulmonary nodules, thus demonstrating its potential for this public health problem. For example, Zhou et al. [32] studied the impact of UHR mode for lung nodule volume evaluation and shape characterization using a PCD-CT system. They used a 512 matrix with a small FOV (11 cm) resulting in a pixel size of 215 µm and compared the UHR mode to the macro mode using two reconstruction algorithms (s80f and b46f). The UHR mode used an effective detector pixel size of 0.25 mm by 0.25 mm at the iso-center, while the conventional macro mode was limited to 0.5 mm by 0.5 mm. For small nodules (diameter $\leq$ 5 mm), UHR mode was able to achieve more accurate volume measurements than macro mode due to higher spatial resolution, which is an advantage for routine use. Moreover, all acquisitions showed comparatively lower bias in the evaluation of the volume of spherical nodules. Additionally, for irregularly shaped (star) nodules, particularly of small size (diameter $\leq$ 5 mm), UHR acquisitions with the sharp kernel provided substantially better accuracy in volume measurements compared to the other three acquisition mode/reconstruction kernel combinations. Furthermore, receiver-operating-characteristics analyses showed a clear benefit of the UHR mode, demonstrating an increased ability to differentiate small, smooth, spherical nodules from small, irregular-shaped nodules. These finding are particularly important, as studies have shown that nodules with irregular or spiculated margins, particularly with distortion of adjacent vessels, are likely to be malignant.

In a second study, Zhou et al. [33] performed a similar study in phantoms with similar parameters and proved that for all nodules, the volume estimation was more accurate, as there was a lower mean absolute percent error (6.5%) compared with macro mode (11.1% to 12.9%). The improvement of volume measurement with the UHR mode was more obvious for small nodule size (3 mm, 5 mm) or star-shaped nodules. Thus, the authors demonstrated that the UHR mode of the evaluated PCD-CT system was able to improve measurement accuracy for nodule volume and nodule shape characterization.

In line with these studies, Kopp et al. [34] demonstrated a better morphological and volumetric evaluation of different nodule phantoms presenting spikes with a different PCD-CT system. The volume estimation indicated better accuracy for PCD-CT compared to CT and HR-CT (with a root mean squared error of 21.3 mm^3 for SPCCT, 28.5 mm^3 for CT, and 26.4 mm^3 for HR-CT). The Dice similarity coefficient was greater for PCD-CT considering all nodule shapes and sizes (mean, PCD-CT 0.90; CT: 0.85; HR-CT: 0.85). These findings were explained by the higher spatial resolution of the system as demonstrated by a higher modulation transfer function (10% modulation transfer function at 21.7 lp/cm).

Recently, using a clinical prototype [22], we demonstrated the enhanced performances of PCD-CT for solid and ground-glass lung nodule detectability in a phantom study using a task-based model observer assessment and a subjective image quality evaluation. The comparison between a dual-layer CT and the PCD-CT system from the same manufacturer with optimized parameters for each platform found a noise reduction with PCD-CT, as demonstrated by the noise power spectrum analysis and an improved spatial resolution as demonstrated by the task transfer function. As a consequence, the task-based model observer (d') evaluation demonstrated a greater detectability for solid and ground-glass nodules (Figure 6). It is noteworthy that the difference in detectability between CT systems was more pronounced for the ground-glass nodules, which are known to be more difficult to detect due to their low contrast with conventional CT systems. Finally, experienced chest radiologists determined that the best compromise for optimal image quality, noise reduction, and increased spatial resolution was reached by using the iterative reconstruction at level iDose 6, which may enable a clinical use.

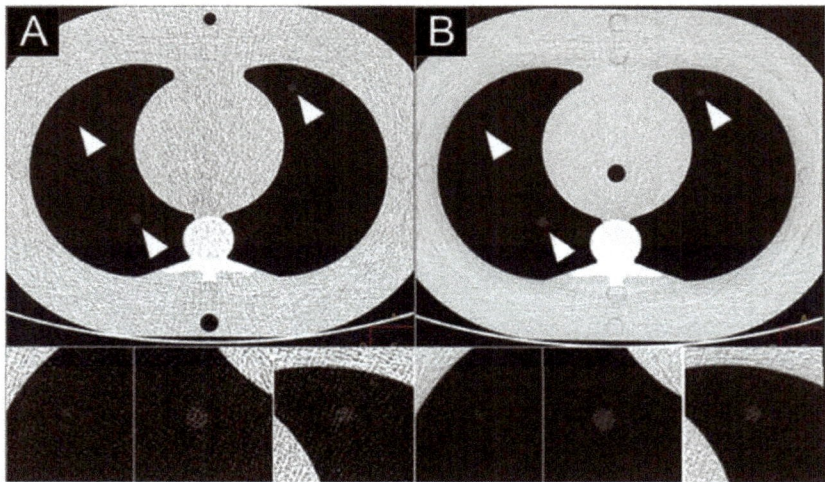

Figure 6. Comparison of high-resolution CT lung imaging of ground-glass nodules (2, 4, 6 mm) between a dual-layer EID-CT (iQon; Philips, Haifa, Israel) (**A**) and a clinical prototype PCD-CT (SPCCT; Philips) (**B**) in an anthropomorphic thorax phantom with an extension ring simulating an obese patient, using a standard dose protocol (120 kVp, 40 mAs).

Finally, Jungblut et al. [35] evaluated the image quality of pulmonary nodule at different low radiation dose for PCD-CT and EID-CT systems. Their analysis was based on a subjective evaluation by observers and on a commercial artificial intelligence-based, computer-aided detection system. They analyzed an anthropomorphic chest phantom containing 14 pulmonary nodules of different sizes with three vendor-specific scanning modes at decreasing matched radiation dose levels. By comparing PCD-CT to EID-CT images, they found using the HR mode a better image quality with PCD-CT in the subjective analysis as well as the lowest image noise in favor of a better objective analysis. Despite the improved performance, the artificial intelligence-based, computer-aided detection system delivered comparable results for lung nodule detection and volumetry between PCD- and dose-matched EID-CT. Nevertheless, the mean sensitivity PCD-CT images was higher than with EID-CT with, for example, a rate of 95% versus 86% for dose-matched EID-CT with a volume CT dose index of 0.41 mGy.

Taken together, these studies show the potential for more accurate lung nodule evaluation in vitro and in vivo with PCD-CT technology that requires confirmation in a prospective clinical study.

3.3. Lung Cancer Screening Imaging

Lung cancer is the leading cause of cancer deaths worldwide [36], and despite the conclusions of the National Lung Screening Trial that CT screening significantly reduces mortality associated with lung cancer, among other diseases [37], to date, there is no worldwide agreement on the screening recommendations. This can in part be explained by the fact that the diagnostic benefits of lung cancer screening have to be balanced with the inherent risks of ionizing radiation as well as overdiagnosis and work-up of false-positive findings [38].

Symons et al. [39] studied the impact of a low-dose acquisition with PCD-CT and a conventional CT with a 512 matrix on two phantoms by comparing attenuation accuracy, noise, and CNR values between different dose settings. Hounsfield unit stability and accuracy for lung, ground-glass nodules, and emphysema were greater with PCD-CT than EID-CT, particularly at lower doses where the attenuation decreased significantly with EID-CT. In addition, a reduction of noise was consistently found for PCD-CT at 80, 100, and 120 kVp in comparison to EID-CT. As a result, CNR were improved compared to EID for ground-glass nodules and emphysema, particularly for 100 and 80 kVp, without significant difference for other objects (acrylic, water, lung foam, air, etc.). These results support the technical benefits of PCD making PCD-CT a promising tool in radiation dose optimization that is critical in further improving the risk-benefit ratio of CT lung cancer screening; however, they require confirmation in a prospective clinical study.

3.4. Low and Ultra-Low Dose Imaging

Ultra-low and low-dose CT has been increasingly used in low-radiation risk assessment of lung cancer, but this is not the only pulmonary disease where the risk-benefit ratio seems positive; for instance, the follow-up of fibrosing disease at low doses of radiation could be of great interest because of the iterative CT scans. However, the main limitation for use of these protocols is the impairment of the objective and subjective image quality because of the photon starvation and increase in artefacts, such as beam hardening using EID-CT. With PCD-CT, numerous studies have suggested an improvement of the image quality (Figures 7 and 8). For instance, Symons et al. [39] proved on phantoms using a 512 matrix the capacity of PCD technology to be more stable in measuring the parenchyma attenuation at low dose. This may also provide better reproducibility and accuracy for quantitative imaging in the future, such as performed for lung density. The latter is necessary to monitor disease, such as alpha-1 antitrypsin deficiency, emphysema, and idiopathic pulmonary fibrosis, but can also be used for the treatment strategy, such as performed in alpha-1 antitrypsin deficiency [40]. More recently, the same group reported in 30 healthy volunteers the feasibility of a CT lung cancer screening protocol (120 kVp, 20 mAs) with a 512 matrix and an iterative reconstruction algorithm [41]. They showed that experienced readers identified the PCD-CT images as having better diagnostic quality for assessment of lung tissue, lung nodules, soft tissue, and bone with lower subjective image noise when compared to those obtained with the EID system. They also found a better image quality in areas with known beam hardening, e.g., around the vertebrae and in the apical lobes. Quantitative measurements showed that PCD-CT images had 15.2–16.8% lower noise at two different dose levels, with 21.0% higher lung nodule CNR. In addition, we demonstrated the feasibility of using low dose (CTDI: 1.11 mGy) and ultra-low dose (CTDI: 0.10 mGy) protocols in lung nodule evaluation with phantoms and one human volunteer while preserving UHR parameters [9]. We used a 1024 matrix, a large FOV, and slice thickness of 0.25 mm and found a satisfactory detection with low X-ray dose protocol for solid, mixed, and ground-glass nodules. Using ultra-low dose parameters (80 kVp, 3 mAs), ground-glass nodules were not clearly defined because of increasing noise. However, iterative reconstruction (i.e., iDose 5 and 9) enabled a satisfactory nodule visualization. Moreover, improved image quality was found with low-dose PCD-CT images compared to standard-dose EID-CT for lung imaging in a human volunteer despite 87% of flux reduction. Additionally, the use of newly developed iterative reconstruction for PCD-CT data led to a decrease in noise by up to 68% when using iDose reconstruction algorithm (iDose 9). In conclusion, this study showed the feasibility of significant dose reduction with PCD-CT with or without iterative reconstruction while conserving the high-resolution parameters for lung analysis.

Taken together, these studies highlight the feasibility of PCD-CT imaging for improving lung nodule detection with a good compromise between increased spatial resolution, decreased dose, and equivalent or reduced noise.

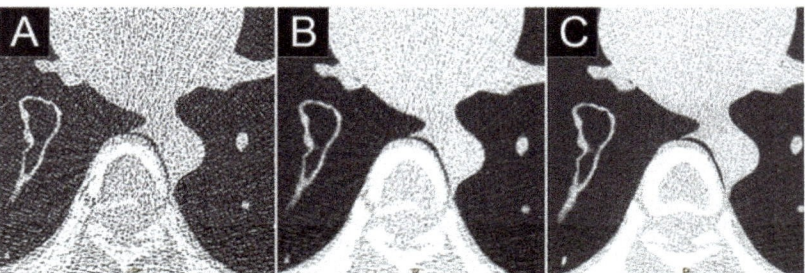

Figure 7. Comparison of high-resolution low dose lung imaging (120 kVp, 10 mAs) between a dual-layer EID-CT (iQon, Philips, Haifa, Israel; (**A**): filter YB, (**B**): filter F) and a clinical prototype PCD-CT (Philips; (**C**): filter detailed 1) in an anthropomorphic phantom CT Torso CTU-41 (Kyoto Kagaku, Tokyo, Japan). Both 1024 matrix and field-of-view of 350 mm were matched. Beam hardening was greatly reduced on the PCD-CT images, greatly improving the image quality.

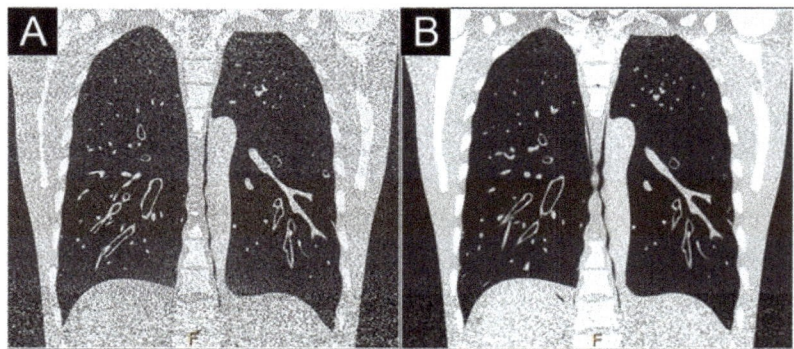

Figure 8. Comparison of high-resolution low dose lung imaging (120 kVp, 10 mAs) between a conventional dual-layer CT (iQon; Philips, Haifa, Israel; (**A**): filter YB) and a clinical PCD-CT (Philips; (**B**): filter detailed 1) in an anthropomorphic phantom CT Torso CTU-41 (Kyoto Kagaku, Tokyo, Japan). Both 1024 matrix and field-of-view of 350 mm were matched. Noise was significantly reduced on the PCD-CT images in the upper and basal lobes, greatly improving the image quality.

3.5. Interstitial Lung Disease Imaging

Interstitial lung diseases are complex pathologies and HR-CT evaluation is essential for accurate diagnosis and determination of the best treatment. However, this requires very high spatial resolution because of the microsemiology of their key signs, e.g., intralobular reticulations, bronchiectasis, and honeycombing, which are frequently indeterminate and may lead to invasive procedures, such as biopsies for histological evaluation [42]. In addition, current low-dose protocols, i.e., lower than 1 mSv, are not recommended due to the impaired image quality that may lead to misclassification of the interstitial lung disease [29]. Therefore, PCD, because of its high resolution and noise reduction capacity, could be a promising tool for ILD evaluation.

In an attempt to evaluate the feasibility of PCD-CT in interstitial lung diseases, a recent study conducted by Ferda et al. [12], with a clinical prototype large FOV PCD-CT system, identified a few cases in a cohort of 60 patients addressed for various reasons. They investigated the diagnostic quality of PCD-CT lung imaging using a standard and a low-dose protocol by subjectively assessing critical structures, such as bronchi and bronchial walls. When PCD-CT images were compared to those obtained with a similar dose using EID-CT, the background noise was significantly lower, and the signal-to-noise ratios were significantly higher in PCD-CT images. An important point is that the subjective quality score between full and low-dose lung imaging was comparable. In patients with interstitial lung disease, the PCD-CT demonstrated a better visualization of higher-order bronchi and third-/fourth-/fifth-order bronchial walls, such as previously suggested with a PCD-CT system from a different manufacturer [9]. However, the authors did not evaluate the diagnostic performance of PCD-CT compared to EID-CT for key signs of fibrosis. Nevertheless, these initial findings indicated an important potential for further radiation dose reduction in interstitial lung disease imaging diagnosis and follow-up.

3.6. Distal Airways and Bronchial Imaging

Bronchial diseases are difficult to evaluate with conventional CT imaging. For patients with chronic obstructive pulmonary disease, the initial morphological evaluation of the bronchial tubes is difficult as well as their follow-up under treatment due to the lack of spatial resolution of conventional scanners. This limitation is also observed for interstitial lung disease, where the differentiation between traction bronchiectasis and honeycombing leads to numerous controversies in the literature [42], leaving a room for image quality improvement using PCD-CT.

For example, Bartlett et al. [30] included 22 patients with pulmonary condition (pneumonia, pulmonary nodule, etc.) and showed improvement in the detection of higher-order bronchi compared with the EID-CT system, irrespective of the image reconstruction kernel used (readers detected more seventh- and eighth-order bronchi). The addition of a sharp reconstruction kernel designed to convey the higher spatial resolution of the PCD-CT system (Q65) further improved the visualization of small bronchi and bronchial walls (walls of the third- and fourth-order bronchi in both lungs). The results of this study demonstrated the potential benefit of PCD-CT lung HR-CT, particularly in assessing airway diseases. Similarly, Kopp et al. [34] compared in-vivo images of a rabbit and a patient acquired with PCD-CT and HR-CT. With HR-CT, bronchi and bronchioles down to a diameter of 1.5–2 mm could be identified. Comparing images of HR-CT and PCD-CT adjusted to the same size, vessels, and walls of bronchioles could be visualized more distinctly with PCD-CT. In addition, we showed a better conspicuity and sharpness of the distal airways as rated by three experienced chest radiologists on a human volunteer, which allowed to see the origin of a 0.5-mm diameter bronchiole that was not visible on an EID-CT [9]. Taken together, these studies support the potential of PCD-CT to propose a new evaluation of bronchial diseases (Figure 9).

3.7. Pulmonary Vascularization Imaging

Pulmonary vascular involvement is highly prevalent in various lung diseases, such as in chronic obstructive pulmonary disease, emphysema, chronic thromboembolic pulmonary hypertension, as well as infectious disease, such as COVID-19 [43–47]. Current standard CT can allow the diagnosis of vessel structure abnormalities, such as thrombus or caliper disparity, while DECT enables the specific imaging of the iodine distribution in the lung, allowing the microcirculation imaging known as a surrogate marker of lung perfusion [48]. Considering the probable improved performance of PCD-CT compared to EID-CT, there is hope for better monitoring the proximal and distal pulmonary vascular involvement in the diseases cited above (Figure 10). For example, this would be of great interest in chronic thromboembolic pulmonary hypertension for the characterization of the involvement of microvasculopathy in the sub-pleural area that might contribute to severe hemodynamics, as suggested by Onishi et al. [49]. In addition, the virtual monoenergetic capabilities of PCD-CT would allow the use of low monoenergetic images, e.g., 40 or 50 keV, to boost iodine attenuation that would help decrease the amount of iodinated contrast agent for a pulmonary CT angiography.

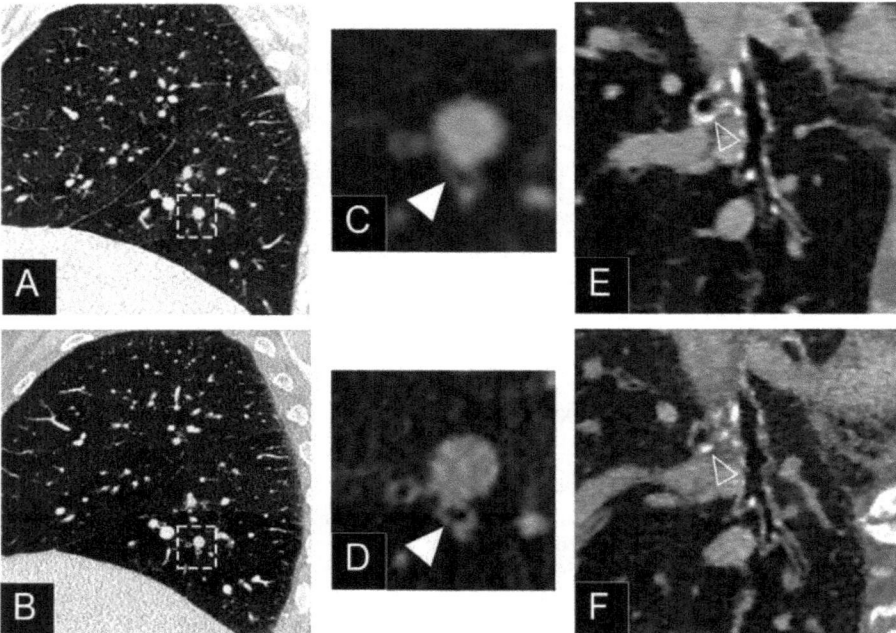

Figure 9. Comparison of the airways imaging in a 72-year-old patient with a respiratory bronchiolitis, which was on the same day as a clinical prototype PCD-CT (first row; Philips, Haifa, Israel) and a dual-layer EID-CT (second row; iQon, Philips). Sagittal views (**A,B**) demonstrated thickening of the bronchial wall as well as a mosaicism probably due to air trapping. Close-up views of the airspaces (**C,D**) showed a better sharpness and conspicuity of the bronchial wall (white arrowheads) with PCD-CT (**D**). Greater sharpness of the bronchial calcifications were noticed on PCD-CT images (**F**) compared to EID-CT images ((**E**); white empty arrowheads).

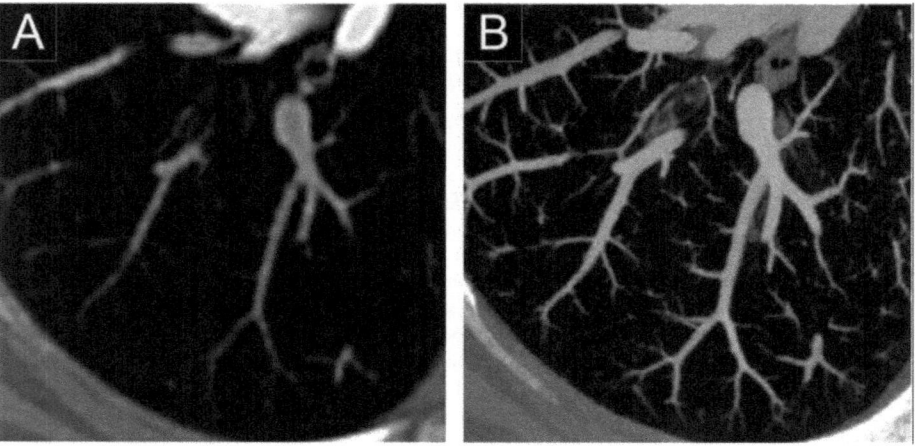

Figure 10. Comparison of the distal arterial pulmonary tree with a dual-layer EID-CT (iQon, Philips, Haifa, Israel; (**A**)) and a clinical prototype PCD-CT (Philips; (**B**)) and) after injection of iodinated contrast agent. The improvement in quality is visible, notably of the distal vessel lumen and calipers that are depicted until the pleural space.

3.8. K-Edge Imaging

Through its multi-energy CT capabilities, PCD technology enables a spectral tissue characterization and differentiation with or without the use of contrast agents, explaining the use of the term spectral photon-counting CT (SPCCT) in recent studies [1,50–66]. Among these capabilities, K-edge imaging is one of the new features of SPCCT enabled by the energy-resolving characteristics of PCD. It is based on the recognition of the specific K-edge signature of an atom, i.e., the binding energy between the inner electron shell and the atom [67]. Indeed, by dividing the spectrum into well-chosen energy-based datasets, it is possible to detect multiple elements, such as gadolinium, gold, and other atoms that have a K-edge within the relevant energy range of the X-ray spectrum used (e.g., ~40–100 keV; Figure 11) [27]. The main advantage of this technique is to permit a specific and quantitative imaging of the agent without any signal arising from the background, which would allow an improved contrast of the tissue as compared to conventional CT imaging. This type of imaging requires the use of contrast agents adapted for SPCCT, which opens the door for research and development. Among the candidate contrast agents for K-edge imaging, nanoparticles are becoming the agents of choice because of their numerous advantages, such as high payload of atoms, potential for blood pool effect, tunable physicochemical properties, potential for targeting imaging, cell tracking, and theranostic applications [50,68,69].

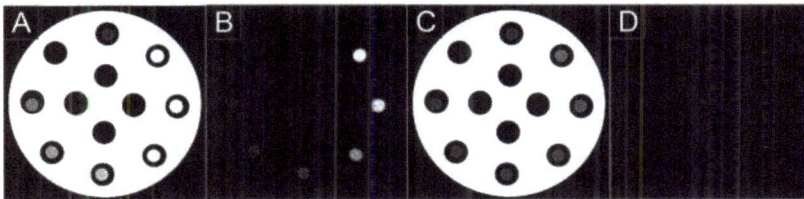

Figure 11. Spectral photon-counting CT (SPCCT) images of a phantom containing tubes with clockwise decrease concentrations of gadolinium from 15 mg/mL to 1 mg/mL of atoms using a clinical prototype (SPCCT; Philips, Haifa, Israel). Conventional image (**A**) and material decomposition of the K-edge image was obtained by reconstructing three material bases (**B**): K-edge image, (**C**): water image, (**D**): iodine image. Only the K-edge images showed the specific signal in the tubes according to the gadolinium concentrations, while water image showed signal from the plastic phantom made of water and the water in the tubes. Iodine image showed no signal accordingly to the absence of iodine.

In 2018 [51], we showed in vitro the feasibility of monocolor and bicolor imaging in order to detect and quantify different mixed contrast agents. Three contrast agents (iodine-, gadolinium-, and gold-based) distributed in tubes at varying proportions were tested by reconstructing the specific images of each material, i.e., based on a two-basis material decomposition (MD) for iodine, three-basis MD for gadolinium or gold with or without iodine, and four-basis MD for gadolinium and gold. The mixtures were prepared such that the solutions could not be differentiated in conventional images. However, distinction was observed in the material images within the same samples, and the measured and prepared concentrations were strongly correlated confirming that SPCCT enables multicolor quantitative imaging in vitro.

Additionally, in 2017 [56], we used a first of its kind system with high-count rate capabilities to demonstrate in vivo in rabbits the feasibility of a dynamic monocolor K-edge imaging of a blood pool agent using PEGylated gold nanoparticles. In the organs analyzed, we showed the persistent visualization of lung vascularization during the first hours after injection. In addition, we presented for the first time the feasibility of bicolor K-edge imaging in animals, i.e., simultaneous differentiation of two different contrast agents, using gold nanoparticles and an iodinated contrast agent (Figure 12). Quantification of these contrast agents in the lungs demonstrated persistent concentration for gold, while for iodine, an arterial first-pass was noticed with rapid clearance in the lungs, as expected. Taken together, these features may potentially allow a new form of functional imaging, where multiple contrast agents with different pharmacokinetics are used simultaneously in the same biological system.

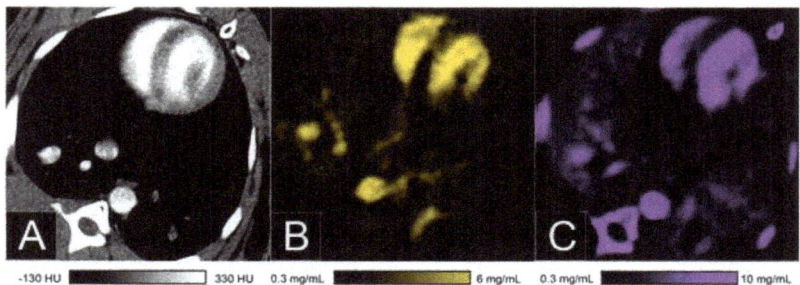

Figure 12. Bicolor imaging of the lung perfusion blood volume in a rabbit after injection of a standard iodinated contrast agent and a contrast agent on a K-edge material (gold nanoparticles) using a spectral photon-counting CT (SPCCT; Philips, Haifa, Israel). Conventional image (**A**) showed the enhancement of the chest vessels as well as the underlying tissue, while the gold K-edge image showed only the signal of gold (**B**). The iodine image showed the signal of iodine as well as misclassification of the bone (**C**).

4. Limitations and Perspectives

The studies cited above provide insight for the future potential of PCD-CT imaging, particularly in-vivo studies that confirm the improvement in spatial resolution and noise management. However, they remain preliminary, and larger patient cohort studies are still needed to identify all the clinical benefits of this new technology. Despite this, it is already possible to consider the clinical potential of SPCCT thanks to studies such as that reported by Yanagawa et al. [70], who proved the value of studying lung adenocarcinomas with a high spatial resolution (2048 matrix on a conventional CT) to define local invasion of the tumor before the surgery.

With respect to the K-edge imaging feature of SPCCT, there are still many hurdles to overcome before considering a clinical translation. These are related to the detection chain and spectral model performance but also by the current contrast agents. It should be noted that, for example, the gadolinium doses needed for in-vivo imaging are far higher than currently used and recommended in MR, and other contrast agents are in an experimental stage that do not allow any kind of clinical human use in the nearer future.

In addition, the current technical limitations of the PCD-CT systems that depend on the progress made by manufacturers should be noted, such as the detector array number, the rotation time, and the energy-resolving capabilities. However, these limitations are expected to be addressed in the near future.

5. Conclusions

Photon-counting detector computed tomography (PCD-CT) represents an emerging medical imaging modality. The key features are an improved spatial and contrast resolution and a significant noise reduction in comparison to the standard energy-integrating detectors CT (EID-CT) as well as spectral capabilities, such as K-edge imaging, that may contribute to the improvement of current CT practice in chest imaging.

Author Contributions: Writing—original draft preparation, S.A.S.-M., J.M. and P.-A.R.; Writing—review and editing, S.B., H.L., V.L., V.C and L.B.; Supervision, S.A.S.-M. and P.D. All authors have read and agreed to the published version of the manuscript.

Funding: This work was supported by European Union Horizon 2020 grant No 668142 and FLI imaging.

Acknowledgments: We are deeply grateful to Philip Robinson for his help in editing the manuscript, Adja Diaw, Daniel Bar-Ness for their help in experiments, Marjorie Villien, Philippe Coulon, Yoad Yagil, Klaus Erhard for their support in the SPCCT project.

Conflicts of Interest: The authors declare no conflict of interest.

References

1. Si-Mohamed, S.; Bar-Ness, D.; Sigovan, M.; Cormode, D.P.; Coulon, P.; Coche, E.; Vlassenbroek, A.; Normand, G.; Boussel, L.; Douek, P. Review of an initial experience with an experimental spectral photon-counting computed tomography system. *Nucl. Instrum. Methods Phys. Res. Sect. A Acce. Spectrometers Detect. Assoc. Equip.* **2017**, *873*, 27–35. [CrossRef]
2. Si-Mohamed, S.; Boussel, L.; Douek, P. Clinical Applications of Spectral Photon-Counting CT. In *Spectral, Photon Counting Computed Tomography: Technology and Applications*; Taguchi, K., Blevis, I., Iniewski, K., Eds.; CRC Press: Boca Raton, FL, USA, 2020; pp. 97–116.
3. Willemink, M.J.; Persson, M.; Pourmorteza, A.; Pelc, N.J.; Fleischmann, D. Photon-counting CT: Technical Principles and Clinical Prospects. *Radiology* **2018**, *289*, 293–312. [CrossRef] [PubMed]
4. Sandfort, V.; Persson, M.; Pourmorteza, A.; Noël, P.B.; Fleischmann, D.; Willemink, M.J. Spectral photon-counting CT in cardiovascular imaging. *J. Cardiovasc. Comput. Tomogr.* **2021**, *15*, 218–225. [CrossRef] [PubMed]
5. Sawall, S.; Amato, C.; Klein, L.; Wehrse, E.; Maier, J.; Kachelrieß, M. Toward molecular imaging using spectral photon-counting computed tomography? *Curr. Opin. Chem. Biol.* **2021**, *63*, 163–170. [CrossRef]
6. Boccalini, S.; Si-Mohamed, S.A.; Lacombe, H.; Diaw, A.; Varasteh, M.; Rodesch, P.-A.; Villien, M.; Sigovan, M.; Dessouky, R.; Coulon, P.; et al. First In-Human Results of Computed Tomography Angiography for Coronary Stent Assessment with a Spectral Photon Counting Computed Tomography. *Investig. Radiol.* **2021**, in press [CrossRef] [PubMed]
7. Taguchi, K.; Iwanczyk, J.S. Vision 20/20: Single photon counting x-ray detectors in medical imaging. *Med. Phys.* **2013**, *40*, 100901. [CrossRef]
8. Blevis, I. X-Ray Detectors for Spectral Photon-Counting CT. In *Spectral, Photon Counting Computed Tomography: Technology and Applications*; CRC Press: Boca Raton, FL, USA, 2020; pp. 179–191.
9. Si-Mohamed, S.; Boccalini, S.; Rodesch, P.-A.; Dessouky, R.; Lahoud, E.; Broussaud, T.; Sigovan, M.; Gamondes, D.; Coulon, P.; Yagil, Y.; et al. Feasibility of lung imaging with a large field-of-view spectral photon-counting CT system. *Diagn. Interv. Imaging* **2021**, *102*, 305–312. [CrossRef] [PubMed]
10. Leng, S.; Rajendran, K.; Gong, H.; Zhou, W.; Halaweish, A.F.; Henning, A.; Kappler, S.; Baer, M.; Fletcher, J.G.; McCollough, C.H. 150-μm Spatial Resolution Using Photon-Counting Detector Computed Tomography Technology: Technical Performance and First Patient Images. *Investig. Radiol.* **2018**, *53*, 655–662. [CrossRef] [PubMed]
11. Da Silva, J.; Grönberg, F.; Cederström, B.; Persson, M.; Sjölin, M.; Alagic, Z.; Bujila, R.; Danielsson, M. Resolution characterization of a silicon-based, photon-counting computed tomography prototype capable of patient scanning. *J. Med. Imaging* **2019**, *6*, 043502. [CrossRef] [PubMed]
12. Ferda, J.; Vendiš, T.; Flohr, T.; Schmidt, B.; Henning, A.; Ulzheimer, S.; Pecen, L.; Ferdová, E.; Baxa, J.; Mírka, H. Computed tomography with a full FOV photon-counting detector in a clinical setting, the first experience. *Eur. J. Radiol.* **2021**, *137*, 109614. [CrossRef] [PubMed]
13. Oostveen, L.J.; Boedeker, K.L.; Brink, M.; Prokop, M.; De Lange, F.; Sechopoulos, I. Physical evaluation of an ultra-high-resolution CT scanner. *Eur. Radiol.* **2020**, *30*, 2552–2560. [CrossRef]
14. Hata, A.; Yanagawa, M.; Honda, O.; Kikuchi, N.; Miyata, T.; Tsukagoshi, S.; Uranishi, A.; Tomiyama, N. Effect of Matrix Size on the Image Quality of Ultra-high-resolution CT of the Lung: Comparison of 512 × 512, 1024 × 1024, and 2048 × 2048. *Acad. Radiol.* **2018**, *25*, 869–876. [CrossRef] [PubMed]
15. Ritschl, L.; Fahrig, R.; Knaup, M.; Maier, J.; Kachelrieß, M. Robust primary modulation-based scatter estimation for cone-beam CT. *Med. Phys.* **2015**, *42*, 469–478. [CrossRef] [PubMed]
16. Pivot, O.; Fournier, C.; Tabary, J.; Letang, J.M.; Rit, S. Scatter Correction for Spectral CT Using a Primary Modulator Mask. *IEEE Trans. Med. Imaging* **2020**, *39*, 2267–2276. [CrossRef]
17. Persson, M.; Huber, B.; Karlsson, S.; Liu, X.; Chen, H.; Xu, C.; Yveborg, M.; Bornefalk, H.; Danielsson, M. Energy-resolved CT imaging with a photon-counting silicon-strip detector. *Phys. Med. Biol.* **2014**, *59*, 6709–6727. [CrossRef] [PubMed]
18. Shikhaliev, P.M. Computed tomography with energy-resolved detection: A feasibility study. *Phys. Med. Biol.* **2008**, *53*, 1475–1495. [CrossRef] [PubMed]
19. Hsieh, S.S. Design considerations for photon-counting detectors: Connecting detectors characteristics to system performances. In *Spectral, Photon Counting Computed Tomography: Technology and Applications*; CRC Press: Boca Raton, FL, USA, 2020; pp. 326–341.
20. Pourmorteza, A.; Symons, R.; Henning, A.; Ulzheimer, S.; Bluemke, D.A. Dose Efficiency of Quarter-Millimeter Photon-Counting Computed Tomography: First-in-Human Results. *Investig. Radiol.* **2018**, *53*, 365–372. [CrossRef] [PubMed]
21. Symons, R.; Reich, D.S.; Bagheri, M.; Cork, T.E.; Krauss, B.; Ulzheimer, S.; Kappler, S.; Bluemke, D.A.; Pourmorteza, A. Photon-Counting Computed Tomography for Vascular Imaging of the Head and Neck: First in vivo human results. *Investig. Radiol.* **2017**, *53*, 135–142. [CrossRef]

22. Si-Mohamed, S.A.; Greffier, J.; Miailhes, J.; Boccalini, S.; Rodesch, P.A.; Vuillod, A.; van der Werf, N.R.; Dabli, D.; Racine, D.; Rotzinger, D.; et al. Comparison of image quality between spectral photon-counting CT and dual-layer CT for the evaluation of lung nodules: A phantom study. *Eur. Rad.* **2021**, in press. [CrossRef] [PubMed]
23. van der Werf, N.R.; Si-Mohamed, S.A.; Rodesch, P.A.; van Hamersvelt, R.W.; Greuter, M.J.W.; Boccalini, S.; Greffier, J.; Leiner, T.; Boussel, L.; Willemink, M.J.; et al. Coronary calcium scoring potential of large field-of-view spectral photon counting CT: A phantom study. *Eur Rad.* **2021**, in press. [CrossRef] [PubMed]
24. Boccalini, S.; Si-Mohamed, S.; Dessouky, R.; Sigovan, M.; Boussel, L.; Douek, P. Feasibility of human vascular imaging of the neck with a large field-of-view spectral photon-counting CT system. *Diagn. Interv. Imaging* **2021**, *102*, 329–332. [CrossRef] [PubMed]
25. Laukamp, K.R.; Lennartz, S.; Neuhaus, V.-F.; Hokamp, N.G.; Rau, R.; Le Blanc, M.; Abdullayev, N.; Mpotsaris, A.; Maintz, D.; Borggrefe, J. Correction to: CT metal artifacts in patients with total hip replacements: For artifact reduction monoenergetic reconstructions and post-processing algorithms are both efficient but not similar. *Eur. Radiol.* **2019**, *29*, 1062. [CrossRef] [PubMed]
26. Do, T.D.; Sawall, S.; Heinze, S.; Reiner, T.; Ziener, C.H.; Stiller, W.; Schlemmer, H.P.; Kachelrieß, M.; Kauczor, H.U.; Skornitzke, S. A semi-automated quantitative comparison of metal artifact reduction in photon-counting computed tomography by energy-selective thresholding. *Sci. Rep.* **2020**, *10*, 21099. [CrossRef]
27. Roessl, E.; Proksa, R. K-edge imaging in x-ray computed tomography using multi-bin photon counting detectors. *Phys. Med. Biol.* **2007**, *52*, 4679–4696. [CrossRef] [PubMed]
28. Webb, W.R. Thin-Section CT of the Secondary Pulmonary Lobule: Anatomy and the Image—The 2004 Fleischner Lecture. *Radiology* **2006**, *239*, 322–338. [CrossRef]
29. Raghu, G.; Collard, H.R.; Egan, J.J.; Martinez, F.J.; Behr, J.; Brown, K.K.; Colby, T.V.; Cordier, J.-F.; Flaherty, K.R.; Lasky, J.A.; et al. An Official ATS/ERS/JRS/ALAT Statement: Idiopathic Pulmonary Fibrosis: Evidence-based Guidelines for Diagnosis and Management. *Am. J. Respir. Crit. Care Med.* **2011**, *183*, 788–824. [CrossRef]
30. Bartlett, D.J.; Koo, C.W.; Bartholmai, B.J.; Rajendran, K.; Weaver, J.M.; Halaweish, A.F.; Leng, S.; McCollough, C.H.; Fletcher, J.G. High-Resolution Chest Computed Tomography Imaging of the Lungs: Impact of 1024 matrix reconstruction and photon-counting detector computed tomography. *Investig. Radiol.* **2019**, *54*, 129–137. [CrossRef]
31. MacMahon, H.; Naidich, D.P.; Goo, J.M.; Lee, K.S.; Leung, A.N.C.; Mayo, J.R.; Mehta, A.C.; Ohno, Y.; Powell, C.A.; Prokop, M.; et al. Guidelines for Management of Incidental Pulmonary Nodules Detected on CT Images: From the Fleischner Society 2017. *Radiology* **2017**, *284*, 228–243. [CrossRef]
32. Zhou, W.; Montoya, J.; Gutjahr, R.; Ferrero, A.; Halaweish, A.; Kappler, S.; McCollough, C.; Leng, S. Lung nodule volume quantification and shape differentiation with an ultra-high resolution technique on a photon-counting detector computed tomography system. *J. Med. Imaging* **2017**, *4*, 043502. [CrossRef]
33. Zhou, W.; Montoya, J.; Gutjahr, R.; Ferrero, A.; Halaweish, A.; Kappler, S.; McCollough, C.; Leng, S. Lung Nodule Volume Quantification and Shape Differentiation with an Ultra-High Resolution Technique on a Photon Counting Detector CT System. *Proc. SPIE Int. Soc. Opt. Eng.* **2017**, *10132*, 101323Q. [CrossRef]
34. Kopp, F.K.; Daerr, H.; Si-Mohamed, S.; Sauter, A.P.; Ehn, S.; Fingerle, A.A.; Brendel, B.; Pfeiffer, F.; Roessl, E.; Rummeny, E.J.; et al. Evaluation of a preclinical photon-counting CT prototype for pulmonary imaging. *Sci. Rep.* **2018**, *8*, 17386. [CrossRef]
35. Jungblut, L.; Blüthgen, C.; Polacin, M.; Messerli, M.; Schmidt, B.; Euler, A.; Alkadhi, H.; Frauenfelder, T.; Martini, K. First Performance Evaluation of an Artificial Intelligence—Based Computer-Aided Detection System for Pulmonary Nodule Evaluation in Dual-Source Photon-Counting Detector CT at Different Low-Dose Levels. *Investig. Radiol.* **2021**, in press. [CrossRef] [PubMed]
36. Jemal, A.; Bray, F.; Center, M.M.; Ferlay, J.; Ward, E.; Forman, D. Global cancer statistics. *CA Cancer J. Clin.* **2011**, *61*, 69–90. [CrossRef] [PubMed]
37. The National Lung Screening Trial Research Team; Aberle, D.R.; Adams, A.M.; Berg, C.D.; Black, W.C.; Clapp, J.D.; Fagerstrom, R.M.; Gareen, I.F.; Gatsonis, C.; Marcus, P.M.; et al. Reduced Lung-Cancer Mortality with Low-Dose Computed Tomographic Screening. *N. Engl. J. Med.* **2011**, *365*, 395–409. [CrossRef] [PubMed]
38. Mayo, J.R.; Aldrich, J.; Müller, N.L. Radiation Exposure at Chest CT: A Statement of the Fleischner Society. *Radiology* **2003**, *228*, 15–21. [CrossRef] [PubMed]
39. Symons, R.; Cork, T.E.; Sahbaee, P.; Fuld, M.K.; Kappler, S.; Folio, L.R.; Bluemke, D.; Pourmorteza, A. Low-dose lung cancer screening with photon-counting CT: A feasibility study. *Phys. Med. Biol.* **2017**, *62*, 202–213. [CrossRef] [PubMed]
40. Green, C.; Parr, D.; Edgar, R.; Stockley, R.; Turner, A. Lung density associates with survival in alpha 1 antitrypsin deficient patients. *Respir. Med.* **2016**, *112*, 81–87. [CrossRef]
41. Symons, R.; Pourmorteza, A.; Sandfort, V.; Ahlman, M.A.; Cropper, T.; Mallek, M.; Kappler, S.; Ulzheimer, S.; Mahesh, M.; Jones, E.C.; et al. Feasibility of Dose-reduced Chest CT with Photon-counting Detectors: Initial Results in Humans. *Radiology* **2017**, *285*, 980–989. [CrossRef] [PubMed]
42. Watadani, T.; Sakai, F.; Johkoh, T.; Noma, S.; Akira, M.; Fujimoto, K.; Bankier, A.A.; Lee, K.S.; Müller, N.L.; Song, J.-W.; et al. Interobserver Variability in the CT Assessment of Honeycombing in the Lungs. *Radiology* **2013**, *266*, 936–944. [CrossRef]
43. Si-Mohamed, S.; Chebib, N.; Sigovan, M.; Zumbihl, L.; Turquier, S.; Boccalini, S.; Boussel, L.; Mornex, J.-F.; Cottin, V.; Douek, P. In vivo demonstration of pulmonary microvascular involvement in COVID-19 using dual-energy computed tomography. *Eur. Respir. J.* **2020**, *56*, 2002608. [CrossRef]
44. Simonneau, G.; Torbicki, A.; Dorfmüller, P.; Kim, N. The pathophysiology of chronic thromboembolic pulmonary hypertension. *Eur. Respir. Rev.* **2017**, *26*, 160112. [CrossRef] [PubMed]

45. Kovacs, G.; Agusti, A.; Barberà, J.A.; Celli, B.; Criner, G.; Humbert, M.; Sin, D.D.; Voelkel, N.; Olschewski, H. Pulmonary Vascular Involvement in Chronic Obstructive Pulmonary Disease. Is There a Pulmonary Vascular Phenotype? *Am. J. Respir. Crit. Care Med.* **2018**, *198*, 1000–1011. [CrossRef] [PubMed]
46. Peinado, V.I.; Pizarro, S.; Barberà, J.A. Pulmonary Vascular Involvement in COPD. *Chest* **2008**, *134*, 808–814. [CrossRef] [PubMed]
47. Iyer, K.S.; Newell, J.D., Jr.; Jin, D.; Fuld, M.K.; Saha, P.; Hansdottir, S.; Hoffman, E.A. Quantitative Dual-Energy Computed Tomography Supports a Vascular Etiology of Smoking-induced Inflammatory Lung Disease. *Am. J. Respir. Crit. Care Med.* **2016**, *193*, 652–661. [CrossRef]
48. Si-Mohamed, S.; Moreau-Triby, C.; Tylski, P.; Tatard-Leitman, V.; Wdowik, Q.; Boccalini, S.; Dessouky, R.; Douek, P.; Boussel, L. Head-to-head comparison of lung perfusion with dual-energy CT and SPECT-CT. *Diagn. Interv. Imaging* **2020**, *101*, 299–310. [CrossRef] [PubMed]
49. Onishi, H.; Taniguchi, Y.; Matsuoka, Y.; Yanaka, K.-I.; Izawa, Y.; Tsuboi, Y.; Mori, S.; Kono, A.; Nakayama, K.; Emoto, N.; et al. Evaluation of microvasculopathy using dual-energy computed tomography in patients with chronic thromboembolic pulmonary hypertension. *Pulm. Circ.* **2020**, *11*, 2045894020983162. [CrossRef] [PubMed]
50. Kim, J.; Bar-Ness, D.; Si-Mohamed, S.; Coulon, P.; Blevis, I.; Douek, P.; Cormode, D.P. Assessment of candidate elements for development of spectral photon-counting CT specific contrast agents. *Sci. Rep.* **2018**, *8*, 12119. [CrossRef] [PubMed]
51. Si-Mohamed, S.; Bar-Ness, D.; Sigovan, M.; Tatard-Leitman, V.; Cormode, D.P.; Naha, P.C.; Coulon, P.; Rascle, L.; Roessl, E.; Rokni, M.; et al. Multicolour imaging with spectral photon-counting CT: A phantom study. *Eur. Radiol. Exp.* **2018**, *2*, 34 [CrossRef] [PubMed]
52. Si-Mohamed, S.; Cormode, D.P.; Bar-Ness, D.; Sigovan, M.; Naha, P.C.; Langlois, J.-B.; Chalabreysse, L.; Coulon, P.; Blevis, I.; Roessl, E.; et al. Evaluation of spectral photon counting computed tomography K-edge imaging for determination of gold nanoparticle biodistribution in vivo. *Nanoscale* **2017**, *9*, 18246–18257. [CrossRef] [PubMed]
53. Si-Mohamed, S.; Thivolet, A.; Bonnot, P.-E.; Bar-Ness, D.; Képénékian, V.; Cormode, D.P.; Douek, P.; Rousset, P. Improved Peritoneal Cavity and Abdominal Organ Imaging Using a Biphasic Contrast Agent Protocol and Spectral Photon Counting Computed Tomography K-Edge Imaging. *Investig. Radiol.* **2018**, *53*, 629–639. [CrossRef] [PubMed]
54. Si-Mohamed, S.; Tatard-Leitman, V.; Laugerette, A.; Sigovan, M.; Pfeiffer, D.; Rummeny, E.J.; Coulon, P.; Yagil, Y.; Douek, P.; Boussel, L.; et al. Spectral Photon-Counting Computed Tomography (SPCCT): In-vivo single-acquisition multi-phase liver imaging with a dual contrast agent protocol. *Sci. Rep.* **2019**, *9*, 8458. [CrossRef]
55. Cormode, D.; Roessl, E.; Thran, A.; Skajaa, T.; Gordon, R.E.; Schlomka, J.-P.; Fuster, V.; Fisher, E.; Mulder, W.; Proksa, R.; et al. Atherosclerotic Plaque Composition: Analysis with Multicolor CT and Targeted Gold Nanoparticles. *Radiology* **2010**, *256* 774–782. [CrossRef] [PubMed]
56. Cormode, D.P.; Si-Mohamed, S.; Bar-Ness, D.; Sigovan, M.; Naha, P.C.; Balegamire, J.; Lavenne, F.; Coulon, P.; Roessl, E.; Bartels, M.; et al. Multicolor spectral photon-counting computed tomography: In vivo dual contrast imaging with a high count rate scanner. *Sci. Rep.* **2017**, *7*, 4784. [CrossRef] [PubMed]
57. de Vries, A.; Roessl, E.; Kneepkens, E.; Thran, A.; Brendel, B.; Martens, G.; Proska, R.; Nicolay, K.; Grüll, H. Quantitative Spectral K-Edge Imaging in Preclinical Photon-Counting X-Ray Computed Tomography. *Investig. Radiol.* **2015**, *50*, 297–304. [CrossRef] [PubMed]
58. Muenzel, D.; Bar-Ness, D.; Roessl, E.; Blevis, I.; Bartels, M.; Fingerle, A.A.; Ruschke, S.; Coulon, P.; Daerr, H.; Kopp, F.K.; et al. Spectral Photon-counting CT: Initial Experience with Dual–Contrast Agent K-Edge Colonography. *Radiology* **2017**, *283* 723–728. [CrossRef]
59. Riederer, I.; Bar-Ness, D.; Kimm, M.A.; Si-Mohamed, S.; Noël, P.B.; Rummeny, E.J.; Douek, P.; Pfeiffer, D. Liquid Embolic Agents in Spectral X-Ray Photon-Counting Computed Tomography using Tantalum K-Edge Imaging. *Sci. Rep.* **2019**, *9*, 5268. [CrossRef]
60. Sigovan, M.; Si-Mohamed, S.; Bar-Ness, D.; Mitchell, J.; Langlois, J.-B.; Coulon, P.; Roessl, E.; Blevis, I.; Rokni, M.; Rioufol, G.; et al. Feasibility of improving vascular imaging in the presence of metallic stents using spectral photon counting CT and K-edge imaging. *Sci. Rep.* **2019**, *9*, 19850. [CrossRef] [PubMed]
61. Thivolet, A.; Si-Mohamed, S.; Bonnot, P.-E.; Blanchet, C.; Képénékian, V.; Boussel, L.; Douek, P.; Rousset, P. Spectral photon-counting CT imaging of colorectal peritoneal metastases: Initial experience in rats. *Sci. Rep.* **2020**, *10*, 13394 [CrossRef] [PubMed]
62. Bratke, G.; Hickethier, T.; Bar-Ness, D.; Bunck, A.C.; Maintz, D.; Pahn, G.; Coulon, P.; Si-Mohamed, S.; Douek, P.; Sigovan, M. Spectral Photon-Counting Computed Tomography for Coronary Stent Imaging: Evaluation of the Potential Clinical Impact for the Delineation of In-Stent Restenosis. *Investig. Radiol.* **2020**, *55*, 61–67. [CrossRef] [PubMed]
63. Boussel, L.; Coulon, P.; Thran, A.; Roessl, E.; Martens, G.; Sigovan, M.; Douek, P. Photon counting spectral CT component analysis of coronary artery atherosclerotic plaque samples. *Br. J. Radiol.* **2014**, *87*, 20130798. [CrossRef] [PubMed]
64. Halttunen, N.; Lerouge, F.; Chaput, F.; Vandamme, M.; Karpati, S.; Si-Mohamed, S.; Boussel, L.; Chereul, E.; Douek, P.; et al. Hybrid Nano-GdF3 contrast media allows pre-clinical in vivo element-specific K-edge imaging and quantification. *Sci. Rep.* **2019**, *9*, 12090. [CrossRef] [PubMed]
65. Riederer, I.; Si-Mohamed, S.; Ehn, S.; Bar-Ness, D.; Noël, P.; Fingerle, A.A.; Pfeiffer, F.; Rummeny, E.J.; Douek, P.; Pfeiffer, D. Differentiation between blood and iodine in a bovine brain—Initial experience with Spectral Photon-Counting Computed Tomography (SPCCT). *PLoS ONE* **2019**, *14*, e0212679. [CrossRef] [PubMed]

66. Si-Mohamed, S.A.; Sigovan, M.; Hsu, J.C.; Tatard-Leitman, V.; Chalabreysse, L.; Naha, P.C.; Garrivier, T.; Dessouky, R.; Carnaru, M.; Boussel, L.; et al. In Vivo Molecular K-Edge Imaging of Atherosclerotic Plaque Using Photon-counting CT. *Radiology* **2021**, *300*, 98–107. [CrossRef] [PubMed]
67. Roessl, E.; Brendel, B.; Engel, K.-J.; Schlomka, J.-P.; Thran, A.; Proksa, R. Sensitivity of Photon-Counting Based K-Edge Imaging in X-ray Computed Tomography. *IEEE Trans. Med. Imaging* **2011**, *30*, 1678–1690. [CrossRef] [PubMed]
68. Hsu, J.C.; Nieves, L.M.; Betzer, O.; Sadan, T.; Noël, P.B.; Popovtzer, R.; Cormode, D.P. Nanoparticle contrast agents for X-ray imaging applications. *Wiley Interdiscip. Rev. Nanomed. Nanobiotechnol.* **2020**, *12*, e1642. [CrossRef]
69. Bouché, M.; Hsu, J.C.; Dong, Y.C.; Kim, J.; Taing, K.; Cormode, D.P. Recent Advances in Molecular Imaging with Gold Nanoparticles. *Bioconjug. Chem.* **2020**, *31*, 303–314. [CrossRef]
70. Yanagawa, M.; Tsubamoto, M.; Satoh, Y.; Hata, A.; Miyata, T.; Yoshida, Y.; Kikuchi, N.; Kurakami, H.; Tomiyama, N. Lung Adenocarcinoma at CT with 0.25-mm Section Thickness and a 2048 Matrix: High-Spatial-Resolution Imaging for Predicting Invasiveness. *Radiology* **2020**, *297*, 462–471. [CrossRef]

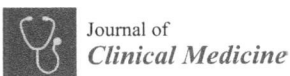

Article

Right Ventricular Volume and Function Assessment in Congenital Heart Disease Using CMR Compressed-Sensing Real-Time Cine Imaging

Benjamin Longère [1,*], Julien Pagniez [2], Augustin Coisne [1], Hedi Farah [2], Michaela Schmidt [3], Christoph Forman [3], Valentina Silvestri [2], Arianna Simeone [2], Christos V Gkizas [2], Justin Hennicaux [2], Emma Cheasty [4], Solenn Toupin [5], David Montaigne [1] and François Pontana [1]

[1] University of Lille, Inserm, CHU Lille, Institut Pasteur Lille, U1011—European Genomic Institute for Diabetes (EGID), F-59000 Lille, France; augustin.coisne@chru-lille.fr (A.C.); david.montaigne@chru-lille.fr (D.M.); francois.pontana@chru-lille.fr (F.P.)

[2] CHU Lille, Department of Cardiovascular Radiology, F-59000 Lille, France; julien.pagniez@chru-lille.fr (J.P.); hedi.farah@chru-lille.fr (H.F.); valentina.silvestri@chru-lille.fr (V.S.); arianna.simeone@chru-lille.fr (A.S.); chgkizas@gmail.com (C.V.G.); justin.hennicaux@chru-lille.fr (J.H.)

[3] MR Product Innovation and Definition, Magnetic Resonance, Siemens Healthcare GmbH, 91052 Erlangen, Germany; michaela.schmidt@siemens-healthineers.com (M.S.); christoph.forman@siemens-healthineers.com (C.F.)

[4] Department of Cardiovascular Imaging, St Bartholomew's Hospital, West Smithfield, London EC1A 7BE, UK; emma.cheasty@nhs.net

[5] Scientific Partnerships, Siemens Healthcare France, 93200 Saint-Denis, France; solenn.toupin@siemens-healthineers.com

* Correspondence: benjamin.longere@chru-lille.fr

Citation: Longère, B.; Pagniez, J.; Coisne, A.; Farah, H.; Schmidt, M.; Forman, C.; Silvestri, V.; Simeone, A.; Gkizas, C.V; Hennicaux, J.; et al. Right Ventricular Volume and Function Assessment in Congenital Heart Disease Using CMR Compressed-Sensing Real-Time Cine Imaging. *J. Clin. Med.* **2021**, *10*, 1930. https://doi.org/10.3390/jcm10091930

Academic Editor: Mickaël Ohana

Received: 16 March 2021
Accepted: 20 April 2021
Published: 29 April 2021

Publisher's Note: MDPI stays neutral with regard to jurisdictional claims in published maps and institutional affiliations.

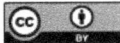

Copyright: © 2021 by the authors. Licensee MDPI, Basel, Switzerland. This article is an open access article distributed under the terms and conditions of the Creative Commons Attribution (CC BY) license (https://creativecommons.org/licenses/by/4.0/).

Abstract: Background and objective: To evaluate the reliability of compressed-sensing (CS) real-time single-breath-hold cine imaging for quantification of right ventricular (RV) function and volumes in congenital heart disease (CHD) patients in comparison with the standard multi-breath-hold technique. Methods: Sixty-one consecutive CHD patients (mean age = 22.2 ± 9.0 (SD) years) were prospectively evaluated during either the initial work-up or after repair. For each patient, two series of cine images were acquired: first, the reference segmented multi-breath-hold steady-state free-precession sequence ($SSFP_{ref}$), including a short-axis stack, one four-chamber slice, and one long-axis slice; then, an additional real-time compressed-sensing single-breath-hold sequence (CS_{rt}) providing the same slices. Two radiologists independently assessed the image quality and RV volumes for both techniques, which were compared using the Wilcoxon test and paired Student's t test, Bland–Altman, and linear regression analyses. The visualization of wall-motion disorders and tricuspid-regurgitation-related signal voids were also analyzed. Results: The mean acquisition time for CS_{rt} was 22.4 ± 6.2 (SD) s (95% CI: 20.8–23.9 s) versus 442.2 ± 89.9 (SD) s (95% CI: 419.2–465.2 s) for $SSFP_{ref}$ ($p < 0.001$). The image quality of CS_{rt} was diagnostic in all examinations and was mostly rated as good ($n = 49/61$; 80.3%). There was a high correlation between $SSFP_{ref}$ and CS_{rt} images regarding RV ejection fraction (49.8 ± 7.8 (SD)% (95% CI: 47.8–51.8%) versus 48.7 ± 8.6 (SD)% (95% CI: 46.5–50.9%), respectively; $r = 0.94$) and RV end-diastolic volume (192.9 ± 60.1 (SD) mL (95% CI: 177.5–208.3 mL) versus 194.9 ± 62.1 (SD) mL (95% CI: 179.0–210.8 mL), respectively; $r = 0.98$). In CS_{rt} images, tricuspid-regurgitation and wall-motion disorder visualization was good (area under receiver operating characteristic curve (AUC) = 0.87) and excellent (AUC = 1), respectively. Conclusions: Compressed-sensing real-time cine imaging enables, in one breath hold, an accurate assessment of RV function and volumes in CHD patients in comparison with standard $SSFP_{ref}$, allowing a substantial improvement in time efficiency.

Keywords: cardiac; heart; magnetic resonance; CMR; compressed sensing; congenital heart disease; GUCH; real-time imaging

1. Introduction

The advent of heart surgery and percutaneous cardiac procedures has considerably improved outcomes in patients born with congenital heart disease [1]. It has led to a growing number of adult survivors with complex congenital heart diseases, with a concomitantly increasing need for imaging follow-up in this clinical context.

Right ventricular (RV) function and volume assessment is of paramount importance in many of these patients, such as in post-repair tetralogy of the Fallot population, as treatment decisions and outcomes mainly rely on RV parameters according to the European Society of Cardiology guidelines for the management of adult congenital heart disease [2]. Although echocardiography remains the first-line investigation, cardiac magnetic resonance (CMR) is a method of choice for RV morphological and functional evaluation in congenital heart disease due to its complex geometry. CMR is considered superior to echocardiography for the evaluation of RV and should be regularly used when the information is essential for patient management, i.e., for quantification of RV volume and ejection fraction, quantification of pulmonary regurgitation, evaluation of RV outflow-tract and pulmonary arteries, detection of myocardial fibrosis or scar, and tissue characterization [2].

However, one major limitation of such extensive CMR examinations is currently the acquisition time, which can be difficult to tolerate in this population, as well as the iterative breath holds, which can be difficult to maintain, leading to poor-quality examinations because of breathing artifacts. To reduce this limitation, the development of acceleration techniques in MR imaging is crucial, and compressed sensing (CS) represents a promising technique in this category. Schematically, CS is a technique that combines a strong and random k-space subsampling, thus enabling a very high scan speed, and it uses non-linear iterative reconstructions to make the final image look as close as possible to that if the k-space had been fully sampled. The use of CS for CMR cine imaging theoretically enables real-time acquisition with whole-ventricle coverage in a single breath hold, and its reliability has been successfully tested in previous studies for left ventricular (LV) or sometimes right ventricular (RV) functional assessment in healthy volunteers and in patients with various extra-congenital pathologies [3–11].

We thus aimed at evaluating the reliability of real-time cine imaging using the CS technique for quantification of RV and LV function and volumes in congenital heart disease patients in comparison with conventional multi-breath-hold segmented steady-state free-precession cine imaging.

2. Materials and Methods

2.1. Study Population

From January to April 2019, 61 consecutive patients were prospectively included. All patients were clinically scheduled for CMR in the context of congenital heart disease for either the initial work-up or after repair. A single-ventricle anatomy was considered as an exclusion criterion. The protocol was approved by our institutional Ethics Committee, and the patients gave informed consent.

2.2. CMR Protocol

All CMR examinations were performed on a 1.5 T magnetic resonance scanner (MAGNETOM Aera, Siemens Healthcare, Erlangen, Germany). For each patient, two series of two-dimensional cine images were systematically acquired: prospectively triggered segmented multi-breath-hold steady-state free-precession sequence ($SSFP_{ref}$) was considered as the reference technique, including a conventional short-axis stack, one LV and one RV two-chamber slice, and one four-chamber slice with an 8 mm slice thickness and a 2 mm gap; an additional prospectively triggered real-time CS sequence (CS_{rt}) in a single breath hold. CS_{rt} cine images were acquired with the same slice number, position, and thickness as those used in the reference technique. An additional phase-contrast imaging sequence was acquired on the pulmonary trunk to assess the RV stroke volume and the severity of the encountered tricuspid regurgitation. The details of the imaging parameters are listed in Table 1.

Table 1. Imaging parameters of the reference steady-state free-precession cine imaging and real-time compressed-sensing cine imaging.

Parameters	SSFP$_{ref}$	CS$_{rt}$
Repetition time—ms	3.16	2.70
Echo time—ms	1.23	1.14
Flip angle—degrees	57	60
Field of view—mm^2	375 × 280	360 × 270
Matrix—pixels^2	288 × 216	224 × 168
Spatial resolution—mm^2	1.3 × 1.3	1.6 × 1.6
Temporal resolution—ms	41.2	49
Slice thickness/gap—mm	8/2	8/2
Bandwidth—Hz/pixel	915	900
ECG mode	Prospective triggering	Prospective triggering
Number of measured cardiac phases per cycle	20 [a]	16 ± 4.1
Reconstructed cardiac frames per cycle—n	20 [a]	20 [b]
Number of views per frame—n	13.0 ± 3.7 [c]	18 [a]
Number of breath holds	13.3 ± 2.9	1 [a]
Cycles of iterative reconstruction—n	NA	40
Breath-hold duration—cardiac cycle per slice	7	2 [d]
Acceleration factor	2	11

Data are expressed as mean ± standard deviation in the absence of any indication. [a] Constant value. [b] Interpolation was performed to provide a constant frame rate of 20 cardiac phases per cycle for post-processing. [c] The number of views per frame was set according to the shorter R–R interval in order to acquire 20 cardiac phases. [d] The first cardiac cycle is required for signal preparation and the second one for signal acquisition. Abbreviations: SSFP$_{ref}$, reference steady-state free-precession cine; CS$_{rt}$, real-time compressed-sensing cine; ECG, electrocardiogram; n, data represented as numbers; NA, not applicable.

2.3. Functional Evaluation

The quantitative assessment consisted of the evaluation of RV functional parameters with both the SSFP$_{ref}$ and CS$_{rt}$ sequences, i.e., ejection fraction (EF), end-diastolic volume (EDV), end-systolic volume (ESV), and stroke volume (SV). The same parameters were measured for the left ventricle, as well as the LV mass. For these quantitative measurements, endocardial and epicardial contours were segmented on the conventional short-axis stacks of cine images using a dedicated analysis software (Cardiac MR analysis workflow, Syngo.via VB30A, Siemens Healthcare, Erlangen, Germany). According to our CMR practice, RV trabeculations were included in the RV volume. Four-chamber and long-axis slices were used as reference images to trace the atrio-ventricular valve planes to ensure an optimal delineation of the heart base for an accurate volume calculation.

2.4. Image Quality Assessment

The overall subjective image quality of the SSFP$_{ref}$ and CS$_{rt}$ cine images was rated on the basis of a four-point Likert scale as follows: 4 = excellent, 3 = good, 2 = fair image quality, and 1 = non-diagnostic examination.

In addition, the objective RV image quality was assessed using previously published criteria, which are mostly based on artifact rating, and they were adapted to the RV [12]. Schematically, 1 point was given if an artifact (fold-over, respiratory ghost, cardiac ghost, image blurring/mistriggering, metallic, or shimming) hampered the visualization of the RV border at the end-systole and/or end-diastole; if such an artifact involved 2 or ≥3 slices, 2 or 3 points were given, respectively.

The depictions of the regional RV wall-motion abnormalities (i.e., hypokinetic, akinetic, or dyskinetic wall) were also rated at 4 anatomical levels (base, mid-cavity, apex, and RV outflow tract), and the depictions of tricuspid-regurgitation-related flow artifacts were assessed on the four-chamber slice.

2.5. Conditions of Image Analysis

The acquired SSFP$_{ref}$ and CS$_{rt}$ cine images were independently analyzed offline by a CMR radiologist (HF) with 3 years of experience. After anonymization, the images from both sequences were randomized and mixed. The two types of cine sequences from one patient were not read in the same session. A radiologist (JP) with 10 years of experience performed the functional RV assessment on a 20-patient sample for the determination of interobserver agreement with the new CS cine technique [13].

2.6. Statistical Analysis

Categorical data are represented as numbers (percentages). Continuous variables are represented as mean ± standard deviation (SD) (95% confidence interval (CI)) in the case of normal distribution and median (range: minimum–maximum) in other cases. SSFP$_{ref}$ and CS$_{rt}$ were compared using paired Student's t test, Bland–Altman, and linear regression analyses. The interobserver agreement of CS$_{rt}$ was determined by calculating the intra-class correlation coefficient. An analysis of variance was performed to compare the RV stroke volumes assessed with both cine sequences with the forward pulmonary volume assessed with PCI. Differences in quality scores between SSFP$_{ref}$ and CS$_{rt}$ were assessed using the Wilcoxon test. Values of $p < 0.05$ were considered statistically significant. For the depictions of valvular regurgitations and wall-motion disorders, a receiver operating characteristic (ROC) curve was used. The statistical analysis was performed with dedicated software (MedCalc 18.11, MedCalc Software bvba, Ostend, Belgium).

3. Results

3.1. Population Description

The 61 patients (29 men, 32 women; mean age: 22.2 ± 9.0 (SD) years; 95% CI: 19.9–24.5 years) underwent CMR for: tetralogy of Fallot ($n = 33/61$; 54.1%), pulmonary atresia with a ventricular septal defect ($n = 7/61$; 11.5%), cardiac shunt ($n = 7/61$; 11.5%), transposition of great arteries ($n = 3/61$; 4.9%), aortic coarctation ($n = 2/61$; 3.3%), congenital pulmonary stenosis ($n = 2/61$; 3.3%), cor triatriatum sinister ($n = 2/61$; 3.3%), congenitally corrected transposition of the great arteries ($n = 2/61$; 3.3%), pulmonary atresia with intact ventricular septum after biventricular repair ($n = 2/61$; 3.3%), and congenital aortic stenosis ($n = 1/61$; 1.6%). Table 2 summarizes further details of the characteristics of the study population.

Table 2. Study population characteristics.

	Mean ± SD (95% CI)	Minimum Value	Maximum Value
Age—years	22.0 ± 9.0 (19.9–24.5)	7	53
Weight—kg	59.1 ± 16.8 (54.8–63.4)	24	100
Height—cm	163.4 ± 15.0 (159.5–167.2)	121	190
Body surface area—m^2	1.6 ± 0.3 (1.6–1.7)	0.9	2.3
Heart rate—beats per minute	74.6 ± 14.2 (71.0–78.2)	44	112

Abbreviations: SD, standard deviation; 95% CI, 95% confidence interval.

3.2. Cine Acquisitions

The mean duration for single-breath-hold CS$_{rt}$ acquisition was 22.4 ± 6.2 (SD) s (95% CI: 20.8–23.9 s) versus 442.2 ± 89.9 (SD) s (95% CI: 419.2–465.2 s) for SSFP$_{ref}$ ($p < 0.001$). The mean acceleration factor provided by CS$_{rt}$ was 20.8 ± 5.6 (95% CI: 19.3–22.2) as compared with SSFP$_{ref}$. A mean number of 13.3 ± 2.9 slices (95% CI: 12.5–14.1 slices) was acquired with each sequence.

3.3. Quantitative Evaluation

Detailed results regarding the SSFP$_{ref}$ and CS$_{rt}$ segmentations for the RV and LV functional parameters are presented in Table 3. There was no statistically significant difference between mean SSFP$_{ref}$ and CS$_{rt}$ for RVEDV (192.9 ± 60.1 (SD) mL (95% CI: 177.5–208.3 mL) versus 194.9 ± 62.1 (SD) mL (95% CI: 179.0–210.8 mL), respectively; $p = 0.169$). The RVEF was slightly underestimated in the CS_{rt} images (CS_{rt}: 48.7 ± 8.6 (SD) % (95% CI: 46.5–50.9%); $SSFP_{ref}$: 49.8 ± 7.8 (SD) % (95% CI: 47.8–51.8%); $p = 0.006$) as a result of a statistically significant but not clinically relevant underestimation of the RVESV in CS_{rt}. The analysis of variance did not demonstrate any significant differences with respect to the RV stroke volume, regardless of the measurement method ($SSFP_{ref}$: 93.6 ± 25.7 (SD) mL (95% CI: 87.0–100.2 mL); CS_{rt}: 92.3 ± 26.0 (SD) mL (95% CI: 85.7–99.0 mL); PCI: 88.6 ± 27.1 (SD) mL (95% CI: 91.6–95.5 mL); $p = 0.605$). No statistically significant differences were visible between $SSFP_{ref}$ and CS_{rt} for LVEF and LVEDV. The LV mass was slightly overestimated in CS_{rt}. The linear regression yielded good agreement between both acquisition techniques for all RV functional parameters (Figure 1), and the r values were excellent for all parameters. On the other hand, graphical analysis of the Bland–Altman plot demonstrated up to five (tetralogy of Fallot, $n = 5/5$; 100%) paired measurements out of the limits of agreement (LOA) depending on the RV parameter considered (LOA in RVEF bias: −13.7 to +9.3%).

Table 3. Functional parameters segmented on both the reference steady-state free-precession and real-time compressed-sensing cine.

	$SSFP_{ref}$ Sequence (mean ± SD (95% CI))	CS_{rt} Sequence (mean ± SD (95% CI))	Mean Difference ± SD (95% CI)	Paired t Test p	ICC Inter	ICC Intra
RVEF—%	49.8 ± 7.8 (47.8–51.8)	48.7 ± 8.6 (46.5–50.9)	−1.07 ± 2.90 (−1.81 to −0.32)	0.006	0.95	0.94
RVEDV—mL	192.9 ± 60.1 (177.5–208.3)	194.9 ± 62.1 (179.0–210.8)	2.00 ± 11.21 (−0.87 to 4.87)	0.169	0.91	0.97
RVESV—mL	98.9 ± 41.0 (88.4–109.4)	102.4 ± 44.0 (91.1–113.7)	3.51 ± 11.05 (0.68–6.34)	0.016	0.97	0.98
RVSV—mL	93.6 ± 25.7 (87.0–100.2)	92.3 ± 26.0 (85.7–99.0)	−1.28 ± 2.96 (−2.04 to −0.52)	0.001	0.99	0.93
LVEF—%	57.4 ± 7.5 (55.4–59.3)	57.8 ± 7.9 (55.7–59.8)	0.38 ± 4.22 (−0.70 to 1.46)	0.488	0.98	0.98
LVEDV—mL	130.0 ± 40.1 (119.8–140.3)	128.7 ± 43.6 (117.5–139.8)	−1.39 ± 10.68 (−4.13 to 1.34)	0.312	0.98	0.97
LVESV—mL	56.3 ± 23.5 (50.3–62.3)	55.5 ± 27.1 (48.5–62.4)	−0.84 ± 10.24 (−3.46 to 1.79)	0.526	0.97	0.98
LVSV—mL	73.6 ± 21.9 (68.0–79.2)	73.4 ± 22.1 (67.7–79.0)	−0.23 ± 3.14 (−1.03 to 0.58)	0.571	0.99	0.99
LVM—g	95.7 ± 33.9 (87.0–104.4)	102.9 ± 38.5 (93.0–112.8)	7.18 ± 15.12 (3.31 to 11.05)	0.0005	0.96	0.97

ICC was used to evaluate the interobserver agreement for the RV segmentation. The significance of Student's t test is defined by $p < 0.05$. Abbreviations: $SSFP_{ref}$, reference steady-state free-precession cine; CS_{rt}, real-time compressed-sensing cine; SD, standard deviation; 95% CI, 95% confidence interval; RV, right ventricular; LV, left ventricular; EDV, end-diastolic volume; ESV, end-systolic volume; SV, stroke volume; LVM, left ventricular mass; ICC, intraclass correlation coefficient; Inter, interobserver; Intra, intraobserver.

3.4. Qualitative Evaluation

Figure 2; Figure 3; Video S1; Video S2 (Supplementary Materials) provide representative examples of the image quality achieved with CS_{rt} images in various clinical situations. The image quality of CS_{rt} was diagnostic in all examinations (Table 4). There was a significantly lower overall image quality score for CS_{rt} images ($p = 0.0001$) because most of the examinations were rated as excellent with $SSFP_{ref}$ and good with CS_{rt}. However, qualitative artifact presence was statistically lower in the CS_{rt} images than in $SSFP_{ref}$ ($p = 0.0016$). Considering $SSFP_{ref}$ as the gold standard, there were no diagnostic losses for regional RV wall-motion abnormalities in CS_{rt} images, demonstrating a 100% sensitivity and specificity (normokinetic: $n = 157/244$ (64.3%); hypokinetic: $n = 39/244$ (16.0%); akinetic: $n = 1/244$ (0.4%); dyskinetic: $n = 47/244$ (19.3%)). The tricuspid-regurgitation-flow void depictions in CS_{rt} images had a sensitivity and specificity of 74.2% and 100%, respectively (predictive positive value = 100%; predictive negative value = 78.9%; area under ROC = 0.87). Using

SSFP$_{ref}$, 23/61 (37.7%) tricuspid regurgitations were depicted (mild: 20/23 (87.0%); moderate: 3/23 (13.0%)). Of the 8/61 (13.1%) tricuspid regurgitations that were not depicted with the CS$_{rt}$ cine, all were quantified as mild with the reference technique (the difference between RVSV and anterograde pulmonary volume was measured with the phase-contrast sequence) [14].

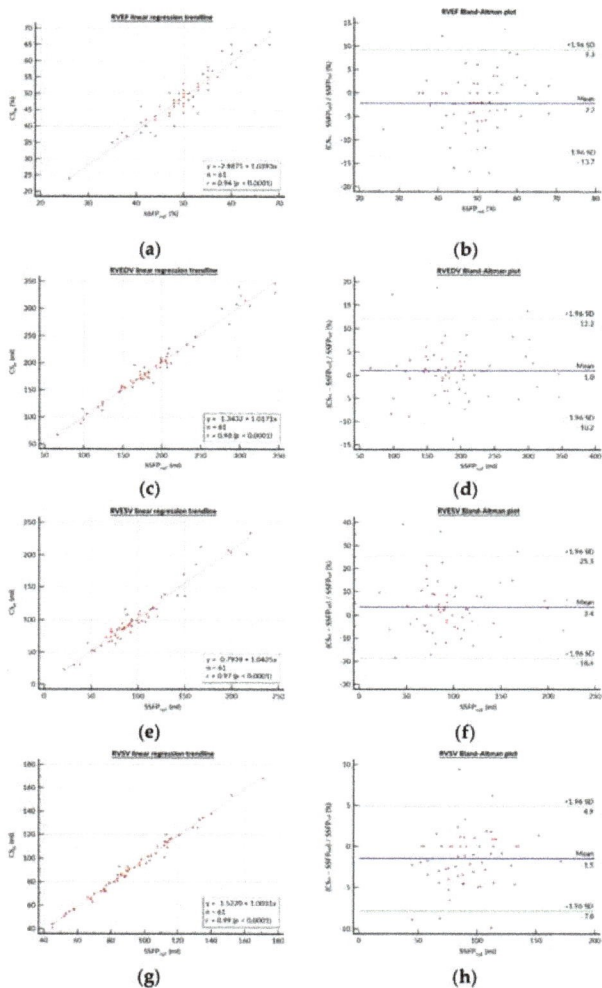

Figure 1. Bland–Altman plots and linear regression trendlines for quantification of the right ventricular functional parameters. Left column: Linear regression trend lines for (**a**) RVEF, (**c**) RVEDV, (**e**) RVESV, and (**g**) RVSV, representing the correlation between parameters measured on the SSFP$_{ref}$ and CS$_{rg}$ sequences. Right column: Bland–Altman plots for the (**b**) RVEF, (**d**) RVEDV, (**f**) RVESV, and (**h**) RVSV. Solid blue lines are the mean differences and dashed green lines are the 95% limits of agreement. Abbreviations: SSFP$_{ref}$, reference steady-state free-precession cine; CS$_{rt}$, real-time compressed-sensing cine; SD, standard deviation; RVEF, right ventricular ejection fraction; RVEDV, right ventricular end-diastolic volume; RVESV, right ventricular end-systolic volume; RVSV, right ventricular stroke volume.

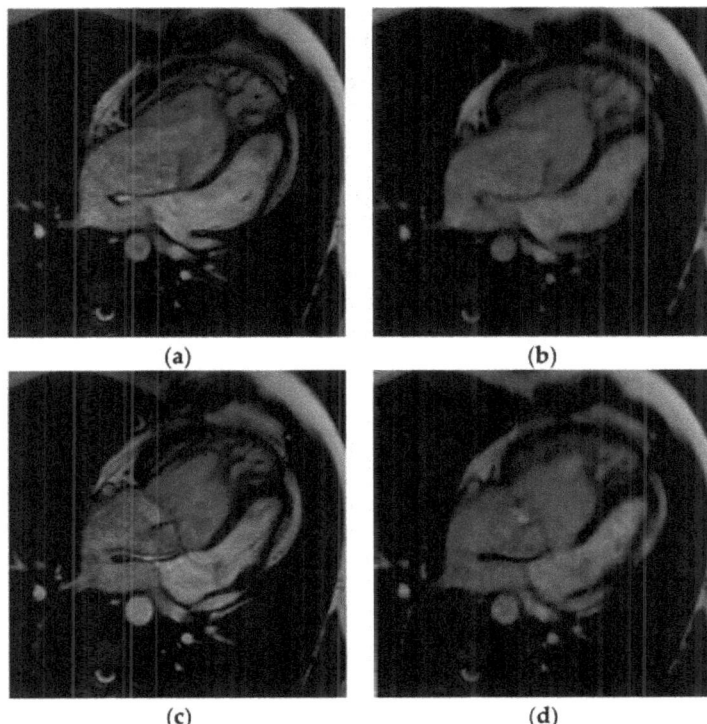

Figure 2. Four-chamber cine slice acquired with both sequences in a 31-year-old male patient referred for transposition of great arteries after a Senning repair follow-up. SSFP$_{ref}$ view in the diastole (**a**) and systole (**c**); overall image quality score = 4/4; RVEF = 42%; EDV = 345 mL. The same slices acquired with CS$_{rt}$ in the diastole (**b**) and systole (**d**); overall image quality score = 3/4; RVEF = 40%; EDV = 346 mL. The tricuspid regurgitation flow artifact remains conspicuous with both sequences (blue arrow). Abbreviations: SSFP$_{ref}$, reference steady-state free-precession cine; CS$_{rt}$, real-time compressed-sensing cine; RVEF, right ventricular ejection fraction; EDV, end-diastolic volume.

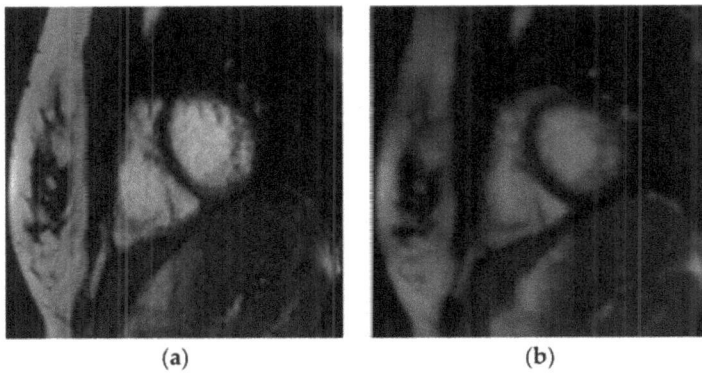

Figure 3. *Cont.*

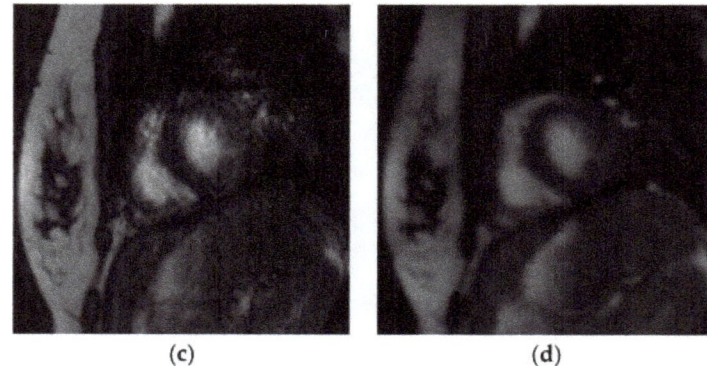

(c) (d)

Figure 3. Short-axis cine slice acquired with both sequences in a 26-year-old female patient referred for a tetralogy of Fallot post-repair follow-up, demonstrating an irregular heart rate. Mean heart rate = 78 ± 14 (SD) bpm (range: 51 to 107 bpm). SSFP$_{ref}$ view in the diastole (**a**) and systole (**c**); overall image quality score = 2/4; RVEF = 51%; EDV = 148 mL. The same slices were acquired with CS$_{rt}$ in the diastole (**b**) and systole (**d**); overall image quality score = 3/4; RVEF = 48%; EDV = 154 mL. The fair image quality is due to the mis-triggering of artifacts in SSFP$_{ref}$, while CS$_{rt}$ provided both accurate segmentation and good image quality. Abbreviations: bpm, beats per minute; SD, standard deviation; SSFP$_{ref}$, reference steady-state free-precession cine; CS$_{rt}$, real-time compressed-sensing cine; RVEF, right ventricular ejection fraction; EDV, end-diastolic volume.

Table 4. Qualitative assessment of the reference steady-state free-precession cine and real-time compressed-sensing cine.

a. Image quality assessment performed for both sequences.							
	Overall image quality score				CMR RV artifact score		
	Score 1 Non-diagnostic	Score 2 Fair	Score 3 Good	Score 4 Excellent	Score 0–3	Score 4–6	Score 7–10
SSFP$_{ref}$—n (%)	1/61 (1.6%)	10/61 (16.4%)	22/61 (36.1%)	28/61 (45.9%)	47/61 (77.1%)	11/61 (18.0%)	3/61 (4.9%)
CS$_{rt}$—n (%)	0/61 (0.0%)	12/61 (19.7%)	49/61 (80.3%)	0/61 (0.0%)	55/61 (90.2%)	6/61 (9.8%)	0/61 (0.0%)
p-value		0.0001				0.0016	

The significance of the Wilcoxon test is defined by $p < 0.05$. Abbreviations: SSFP$_{ref}$, reference steady-state free-precession cine; CS$_{rt}$, real-time compressed-sensing cine; n (%), data represented as numbers (percentages); CMR, cardiac magnetic resonance; RV, right ventricle.

b. Diagnostic performance crosstabulation for tricuspid-regurgitation-flow-related artifact depiction.			
	SSFP$_{ref}$: TR+	SSFP$_{ref}$: TR−	Total
CS$_{rt}$: TR+	23/61 (37.7%)	0 (0.0%)	23/61 (37.7%)
CS$_{rt}$: TR−	8/61 (13.1%)	30 (49.2%)	38/61 (62.3%)
Total	31/61 (50.8%)	30/61 (49.2%)	61/61 (100.0%)

Considering SSFP$_{ref}$ as the gold standard, CS$_{rt}$ demonstrated the following diagnostic performances for the depiction of tricuspid-regurgitation-flow-related artifacts: sensitivity = 74.2%; specificity = 100%; positive predictive value = 100%; negative predictive value = 78.9%; area under ROC = 0.87. Abbreviations: SSFP$_{ref}$, reference steady-state free-precession cine; CS$_{rt}$, real-time compressed-sensing cine; TR+, conspicuous tricuspid-regurgitation-flow-related artifact; TR−, no tricuspid-regurgitation-flow-related artifact depicted; ROC, receiver operating characteristic.

4. Discussion

Our prospective monocentric study based on a cohort of 61 pediatric and grown-up CHD patients, including 33 tetralogies of Fallot, demonstrated that the quantification of RV function and volumes yields similar results for CS$_{rt}$ and for the standard SSFP$_{ref}$ cine techniques, while the former allows a drastically shorter acquisition time. The agreement between CS$_{rt}$ and SSFP$_{ref}$ regarding the RV volume assessment is in line with the findings of previous studies performed on smaller cohorts of healthy volunteers and non-CHD patients [5,10]. The *t* test comparisons performed in our study demonstrated a statistically significant trend towards a 1.07% RVEF underestimation (relative mean difference = −2.14%), a 3.51 mL RVESV overestimation (relative mean difference = 3.54%), and a 1.28 mL RVSV underestimation (relative mean difference = −1.36%) with CS$_{rt}$. The segmented steady-state free precession cine is currently considered the gold-standard technique for the measurement of ventricular volumes, including in CHD patients [2,15–17]. However, these trends must be balanced with the clinically relevant LOA demonstrated in the Bland–Altman plots, mainly regarding the relative bias of RVEF (−13.7; +9.3%), which was also the case in other studies evaluating CS cine for RV assessment in non-CHD populations, where the LOA was reported to be from −10.5 to +11.6% [5,10,18,19]. A more recent study also found a similar performance of a novel real-time steady-state free precession spiral sequence reconstructed using CS in a pediatric-only CHD population, but did not evaluate the regional wall-motion abnormalities or the depiction of tricuspid-regurgitation-related flow artifacts [19]. It must also be highlighted that both intra- and interobserver agreement was excellent for all CS_{rt}-evaluated RV functional parameters. Additionally, our findings demonstrate a strong agreement between both $SSFP_{ref}$ and CS_{rt} for functional LV parameters, despite the slight LV mass overestimation with CS_{rt}, as previously reported [5].

The best image plane required for post-processing of RV volumes has long been debated, especially in the clinical context of CHD. However, it has been shown that despite a trend favoring the axial plane rather than the short axis in terms of reproducibility, there were no clinically significant differences between these two contouring methods [20]. Thus, we drew RV endocardial contours on short-axis stacks, as this is widely performed and is easier to set up in routine practice, but care was taken to trace the tricuspid valve on reference four-chamber and RV long-axis slices to delimit the right ventricular basis as precisely as possible. Despite controversies about segmentation methods, we included trabeculations in RV volumes according to our CMR center's habits [21]. The justification for this choice lies in the need for consistency in our practice in order to preserve reproducibility in patient follow-ups [22,23]. Nevertheless, we acknowledge that excluding trabeculations from the blood volume could be more accurate [24]. This could explain the lower dispersion of the differences in parameters measured with $SSFP_{ref}$ and CS_{rt} on Bland–Altman plots when the RVEF or RVESV increase (Figure 1b,h).

The CS_{rt} images were diagnostic in all examinations, but the overall image quality score was, as expected, significantly lower with this technique. This can be explained by the lower edge definition provided by CS, which resulted in a slightly blurry aspect of the images. This should be addressed by using a two-shot variant of the evaluated compressed-sensing cine, which would provide an improved edge sharpness and would preserve the important scan time reduction [25]. Nevertheless, this two-shot variant has not yet been evaluated for the right ventricular functional parameters and should be the subject of further study. However, a lower RV artifact score was found with CS_{rt} due to the reduction of artifacts—which were mostly related to mis-triggering—achieved with this real-time acquisition technique. In addition, the performance of CS_{rt} for RV wall-motion disorder depiction was very high, as there was no diagnostic loss in comparison with the reference images, and only mild tricuspid regurgitations were not depicted with CS_{rt} cine (Figure 2; Video S1 (Supplementary Materials)). These findings are in line with a recently published study evaluating the same real-time CS cine sequences for both LV and RV assessment in a non-selected adult cohort [18].

The CS_{rt} sequence consisted of a single-breath-hold cine acquisition; however, some patients could not fully achieve the required apnea due to their clinical condition. They were not excluded from the study, as our aim was to be as representative as possible of our CHD population that we encounter in daily practice. Despite these free-breathing ends of acquisition, no major artifacts (CMR RV quality score > 7/10) were noticed in the CS_{rt} images, which all had diagnostic quality. These findings strongly suggest the possibility of the free-breathing acquisition of CS_{rt} cine, which is particularly relevant for pediatric or end-stage CHD patients. Although the aim of this study was not to evaluate free-breathing imaging protocol, free-breathing CS_{rt} has been demonstrated to be a reliable alternative that allows faster acquisition than sequences based on registration of multiple acquisitions and motion-correction algorithms [9,26]. The acceleration provided by CS_{rt} may allow one to either (a) shorten breath-holding duration by splitting the stacks of cine slices to reduce the number of cine loops acquired per breath hold, especially for patients with shortness of breath, or (b) to shorten the overall examination duration, as suggested in the present study (average: 22 s (CS_{rt}) versus 7 min and 22 s ($SSFP_{ref}$) for 13 cine slices) to improve the clinical workflow and tolerance in children or to spare examination time in order to acquire additional sequences. Indeed, a comprehensive study of hemodynamic patterns is a key point in the initial work-up of CHD or in repair follow-up. Four-dimensional (4D) flow is a promising but time-consuming technique that may take advantage of the thusly spared time [27,28]. Depending on the sequence design, this technique may provide both qualitative and quantitative assessments of flow patterns and ventricular volumes [29]. As extended examination durations are an obstacle for the routine use of 4D flow, compressed-sensing 4D flow prototypes are also being developed [30–32].

Another interesting point is the decrease in the mis-triggering artifacts observed with CS_{rt} (Figure 3; Video S2 (Supplementary Materials)). Even though it was not the purpose of our study and would require further dedicated studies, this finding suggests that CS_{rt} might have an important part to play for functional or WMD evaluations in patients with irregular heart rates [33].

Limitations

The minimum age in our population was 7 years, and further studies would be needed for validation in younger children. We also have to report that despite the drastic decrease in acquisition time, the data reconstruction process was more time consuming than with $SSFP_{ref}$, as 2 min were necessary in order to visualize the whole cine stack in spite of a graphics processing unit upgrade.

Regarding the blurry aspect of images that we observed with CS, it must be said that the CS_{rt} sequence was designed in order to reduce the acquisition time as much as possible. In a different way, some authors have successfully tested CS cine to improve the spatial or temporal resolution with quite similar or even moderately shorter acquisition times than those for reference $SSFP_{ref}$, or even to achieve three-dimensional cine acquisitions [34–36]. Our scan time was, however, strongly reduced, as low as 22.4 ± 6.2 (SD) s versus about 6 to 10 min for segmented multi-breath-hold $SSFP_{ref}$, which can be very useful for patient comfort and workflow.

Although it is in line with the current literature, the bias observed between the two sequences in RVEF measurement (~10%) is clinically relevant and must be taken into consideration in CHD follow-up [37,38]. The reason for such a bias may lie in the edge sharpness impairment induced by CS_{rt} as compared to $SSFP_{ref}$ [18]. Indeed, the partial Fourier and the interpolation performed to provide a constant cardiac frame rate for post-processing induced a smoother and blurrier endocardial delineation than conventional cine. This limitation should be responsible for the increased bias in segmentation between the two techniques and may be solved by a multi-shot approach to CS acceleration [25].

5. Conclusions

Compressed-sensing real-time cine imaging enables the assessment RV function and volumes in patients with CHD while providing a significant reduction in examination duration and allowing an improvement in time efficiency and patient care.

Supplementary Materials: The following are available online at https://www.mdpi.com/article/10.3390/jcm10091930/s1, Video S1: Four-chamber cine slice in a 31-year-old male patient referred for transposition of great arteries after a Senning repair (same patient as Figure 2); Video S2: Four-chamber cine slice in a 27-year-old female patient referred for tetralogy of Fallot follow-up.

Author Contributions: B.L.: data collection, interpretation and analysis, drafting of the manuscript, critical revision for important intellectual content; J.P.: study conception and design, data collection, interpretation and analysis, drafting of the manuscript, critical revision for important intellectual content; A.C.: study conception, critical revision for important intellectual content; H.F.: data collection, interpretation and analysis, drafting of the manuscript; M.S.: study conception and design, critical revision for important intellectual content; C.F.: study conception and design, critical revision for important intellectual content; V.S.: data collection and interpretation, critical revision for important intellectual content; A.S.: data collection and interpretation, critical revision for important intellectual content; C.V.G.: data collection and interpretation, critical revision for important intellectual content; J.H.: data collection and interpretation, critical revision for important intellectual content. E.C.: study conception, critical revision for important intellectual content; S.T.: study conception and design, critical revision for important intellectual content; D.M.: study conception, critical revision for important intellectual content; F.P.: study conception and design, data collection, interpretation and analysis, drafting of the manuscript, critical revision for important intellectual content. All authors have read and agreed to the published version of the manuscript.

Funding: This research received no external funding.

Institutional Review Board Statement: The study was approved by the research ethics committee of Lille University Hospital.

Informed Consent Statement: Informed consent was obtained from all subjects involved in the study.

Data Availability Statement: The data presented in this study are available on reasonable request from the corresponding author, subject to approval by the research ethics committee of Lille University Hospital.

Conflicts of Interest: B.L., J.P., A.C., H.F., V.S., A.S., C.V.G., J.H., E.C., D.M., and F.P. have no competing interests. They are employed by an institution engaged in a contractual collaboration with Siemens Healthcare. M.S., C.F., and S.T. are employees of Siemens Healthcare GmbH.

References

1. Khairy, P.; Ionescu-Ittu, R.; Mackie, A.S.; Abrahamowicz, M.; Pilote, L.; Marelli, A.J. Changing Mortality in Congenital Heart Disease. *J. Am. Coll. Cardiol.* **2010**, *56*, 1149–1157. [CrossRef] [PubMed]
2. Baumgartner, H.; De Backer, J.; Babu-Narayan, S.V.; Budts, W.; Chessa, M.; Diller, G.-P.; Lung, B.; Kluin, J.; Lang, I.M.; Meijboom, F.; et al. 2020 ESC Guidelines for the Management of Adult Congenital Heart Disease. *Eur. Heart J.* **2021**, *42*, 563–645. [CrossRef]
3. Vincenti, G.; Monney, P.; Chaptinel, J.; Rutz, T.; Coppo, S.; Zenge, M.O.; Schmidt, M.; Nadar, M.S.; Piccini, D.; Chèvre, P.; et al. Compressed Sensing Single-Breath-Hold CMR for Fast Quantification of LV Function, Volumes, and Mass. *J. Am. Coll. Cardiol. Imaging* **2014**, *7*, 882–892. [CrossRef] [PubMed]
4. Kido, T.; Kido, T.; Nakamura, M.; Watanabe, K.; Schmidt, M.; Forman, C.; Mochizuki, T. Compressed Sensing Real-Time Cine Cardiovascular Magnetic Resonance: Accurate Assessment of Left Ventricular Function in a Single-Breath-Hold. *J. Cardiovasc. Magn. Reson.* **2016**, *18*, 50–60. [CrossRef]
5. Sudarski, S.; Henzler, T.; Haubenreisser, H.; Dösch, C.; Zenge, M.O.; Schmidt, M.; Nadar, M.S.; Borggrefe, M.; Schoenberg, S.O.; Papavassiliu, T. Free-Breathing Sparse Sampling Cine MR Imaging with Iterative Reconstruction for the Assessment of Left Ventricular Function and Mass at 3.0 T. *Radiology* **2017**, *282*, 74–83. [CrossRef]
6. Allen, B.D.; Carr, M.; Botelho, M.P.F.; Rahsepar, A.A.; Markl, M.; Zenge, M.O.; Schmidt, M.; Nadar, M.S.; Spottiswoode, B.; Collins, J.D.; et al. Highly Accelerated Cardiac MRI Using Iterative SENSE Reconstruction: Initial Clinical Experience. *Int. J. Cardiovasc. Imaging* **2016**, *32*, 955–963. [CrossRef] [PubMed]
7. Camargo, G.C.; Erthal, F.; Sabioni, L.; Penna, F.; Strecker, R.; Schmidt, M.; Zenge, M.O.; Lima, R.d.S.L.; Gottlieb, I. Real-Time Cardiac Magnetic Resonance Cine Imaging with Sparse Sampling and Iterative Reconstruction for Left-Ventricular Measures: Comparison with Gold-Standard Segmented Steady-State Free Precession. *Magn. Reson. Imaging* **2017**, *38*, 138–144. [CrossRef] [PubMed]
8. Goebel, J.; Nensa, F.; Bomas, B.; Schemuth, H.P.; Maderwald, S.; Gratz, M.; Quick, H.H.; Schlosser, T.; Nassenstein, K. Real-Time SPARSE-SENSE Cardiac Cine MR Imaging: Optimization of Image Reconstruction and Sequence Validation. *Eur. Radiol.* **2016**, *26*, 4482–4489. [CrossRef] [PubMed]
9. Kido, T.; Kido, T.; Nakamura, M.; Watanabe, K.; Schmidt, M.; Forman, C. Mochizuki, T. Assessment of Left Ventricular Function and Mass on Free-Breathing Compressed Sensing Real-Time Cine Imaging. *Circ. J.* **2017**, *81*, 1463–1468. [CrossRef]
10. Bogachkov, A.; Ayache, J.B.; Allen, B.D.; Murphy, I.; Carr, M.L.; Spottiswoode, B.; Schmidt, M.; Zenge, M.O.; Nadar, M.S.; Zuehlsdorff, S.; et al. Right Ventricular Assessment at Cardiac MRI: Initial Clinical Experience Utilizing an IS-SENSE Reconstruction. *Int. J. Cardiovasc. Imaging* **2016**, *32*, 1081–1091. [CrossRef] [PubMed]
11. Haubenreisser, H.; Henzler, T.; Budjan, J.; Sudarski, S.; Zenge, M.O.; Schmidt, M.; Nadar, M.S.; Borggrefe, M.; Schoenberg, S.O.; Papavassiliu, T. Right Ventricular Imaging in 25 Seconds: Evaluating the Use of Sparse Sampling CINE with Iterative Reconstruction for Volumetric Analysis of the Right Ventricle. *Investig. Radiol.* **2016**, *51*, 379–386. [CrossRef]
12. Klinke, V.; Muzzarelli, S.; Lauriers, N.; Locca, D.; Vincenti, G.; Monney, P.; Lu, C.; Nothnagel, D.; Pilz, G.; Lombardi, M.; et al. Quality Assessment of Cardiovascular Magnetic Resonance in the Setting of the European CMR Registry: Description and Validation of Standardized Criteria. *J. Cardiovasc. Magn. Reson.* **2013**, *15*, 55. [CrossRef]
13. Benchoufi, M.; Matzner-Lober, E.; Molinari, N.; Jannot, A.-S.; Soyer, P. Interobserver Agreement Issues in Radiology. *Diagn. Interv. Imaging* **2020**, *101*, 639–641. [CrossRef] [PubMed]

14. Myerson, S.G. Valvular and Hemodynamic Assessment with CMR. *Heart Fail. Clin.* **2009**, *5*, 389–400. [CrossRef] [PubMed]
15. Plein, S.; Bloomer, T.N.; Ridgway, J.P.; Jones, T.R.; Bainbridge, G.J.; Sivananthan, M.U. Steady-State Free Precession Magnetic Resonance Imaging of the Heart: Comparison with Segmented k-Space Gradient-Echo Imaging. *J. Magn. Reson. Imaging* **2001**, *14*, 230–236. [CrossRef] [PubMed]
16. Pennell, D.J.; Sechtem, U.P.; Higgins, C.B.; Manning, W.J.; Pohost, G.M.; Rademakers, F.E.; van Rossum, A.C.; Shaw, L.J.; Yucel, E.K.; Society for Cardiovascular Magnetic Resonance; et al. Clinical Indications for Cardiovascular Magnetic Resonance (CMR): Consensus Panel Report. *Eur. Heart J.* **2004**, *25*, 1940–1965. [CrossRef]
17. Kramer, C.M.; Barkhausen, J.; Bucciarelli-Ducci, C.; Flamm, S.D.; Kim, R.J.; Nagel, E. Standardized Cardiovascular Magnetic Resonance Imaging (CMR) Protocols: 2020 Update. *J. Cardiovasc. Magn. Reson.* **2020**, *22*, 17. [CrossRef]
18. Vermersch, M.; Longère, B.; Coisne, A.; Schmidt, M.; Forman, C.; Monnet, A.; Pagniez, J.; Silvestri, V.; Simeone, A.; Cheasty, E.; et al. Compressed Sensing Real-Time Cine Imaging for Assessment of Ventricular Function, Volumes and Mass in Clinical Practice. *Eur. Radiol.* **2020**, *30*, 609–619. [CrossRef]
19. Steeden, J.A.; Kowalik, G.T.; Tann, O.; Hughes, M.; Mortensen, K.H.; Muthurangu, V. Real-Time Assessment of Right and Left Ventricular Volumes and Function in Children Using High Spatiotemporal Resolution Spiral BSSFP with Compressed Sensing. *J. Cardiovasc. Magn. Reson.* **2018**, *20*, 79. [CrossRef]
20. Clarke, C.J.; Gurka, M.J.; Norton, P.T.; Kramer, C.M.; Hoyer, A.W. Assessment of the Accuracy and Reproducibility of RV Volume Measurements by CMR in Congenital Heart Disease. *J. Am. Coll. Cardiol. Imaging* **2012**, *5*, 28–37. [CrossRef]
21. Schulz-Menger, J.; Bluemke, D.A.; Bremerich, J.; Flamm, S.D.; Fogel, M.A.; Friedrich, M.G.; Kim, R.J.; von Knobelsdorff-Brenkenhoff, F.; Kramer, C.M.; Pennell, D.J.; et al. Standardized Image Interpretation and Post-Processing in Cardiovascular Magnetic Resonance—2020 Update. *J. Cardiovasc. Magn. Reson.* **2020**, *22*, 19. [CrossRef]
22. Winter, M.M.; Bernink, F.J.; Groenink, M.; Bouma, B.J.; van Dijk, A.P.; Helbing, W.A.; Tijssen, J.G.; Mulder, B.J. Evaluating the Systemic Right Ventricle by CMR: The Importance of Consistent and Reproducible Delineation of the Cavity. *J. Cardiovasc. Magn. Reson.* **2008**, *10*, 40. [CrossRef] [PubMed]
23. Fratz, S.; Chung, T.; Greil, G.F.; Samyn, M.M.; Taylor, A.M.; Valsangiacomo Buechel, E.R.; Yoo, S.-J.; Powell, A.J. Guidelines and Protocols for Cardiovascular Magnetic Resonance in Children and Adults with Congenital Heart Disease: SCMR Expert Consensus Group on Congenital Heart Disease. *J. Cardiovasc. Magn. Reson.* **2013**, *15*, 51. [CrossRef] [PubMed]
24. Bonello, B.; Kilner, P.J. Review of the Role of Cardiovascular Magnetic Resonance in Congenital Heart Disease, with a Focus on Right Ventricle Assessment. *Arch. Cardiovasc. Dis.* **2012**, *105*, 605–613. [CrossRef] [PubMed]
25. Wang, J.; Li, X.; Lin, L.; Dai, J.-W.; Schmidt, M.; Forman, C.; An, J.; Jin, Z.-Y.; Wang, Y.-N. Diagnostic Efficacy of 2-Shot Compressed Sensing Cine Sequence Cardiovascular Magnetic Resonance Imaging for Left Ventricular Function. *Cardiovasc. Diagn. Ther.* **2020**, *10*, 431–441. [CrossRef] [PubMed]
26. Kellman, P.; Chefd'hotel, C.; Lorenz, C.H.; Mancini, C.; Arai, A.E.; McVeigh, E.R. High Spatial and Temporal Resolution Cardiac Cine MRI from Retrospective Reconstruction of Data Acquired in Real Time Using Motion Correction and Resorting. *Magn. Reson. Med.* **2009**, *62*, 1557–1564. [CrossRef]
27. Rizk, J. 4D Flow MRI Applications in Congenital Heart Disease. *Eur. Radiol.* **2021**, *31*, 1160–1174. [CrossRef] [PubMed]
28. Gabiano, E.; Silvestri, V.; Pagniez, J.; Simeone, A.; Hennicaux, J.; Longere, B.; Pontana, F. Le flux 4D: Technique et principales applications pour l'étude de l'aorte thoracique. *J. Imaging Diagn. Interv.* **2020**. [CrossRef]
29. Barker, N.; Fidock, B.; Johns, C.S.; Kaur, H.; Archer, G.; Rajaram, S.; Hill, C.; Thomas, S.; Karunasaagarar, K.; Capener, D.; et al. A Systematic Review of Right Ventricular Diastolic Assessment by 4D Flow CMR. *BioMed Res. Int.* **2019**, *2019*. [CrossRef]
30. Tariq, U.; Hsiao, A.; Alley, M.; Zhang, T.; Lustig, M.; Vasanawala, S.S. Venous and Arterial Flow Quantification Are Equally Accurate and Precise with Parallel Imaging Compressed Sensing 4D Phase Contrast MRI. *J. Magn. Reson. Imaging* **2013**, *37*, 1419–1426. [CrossRef]
31. Longere, B.; Braye, G.; Pagniez, J.; Silvestri, V.; Simeone, A.; Kasprzak, K.; Monnet, A.; Pontana, F. Compressed Sensing 4D Flow MRI for the Assessment of the Left Ventricular Stroke Volume. In Proceedings of the European Society of Cardiovascular Radiology Congress, Antwerp, Belgium, 24–26 October 2019; p. P-0047.
32. Hsiao, A.; Lustig, M.; Alley, M.T.; Murphy, M.; Chan, F.P.; Herfkens, R.J.; Vasanawala, S.S. Rapid Pediatric Cardiac Assessment of Flow and Ventricular Volume with Compressed Sensing Parallel Imaging Volumetric Cine Phase-Contrast MRI. *Am. J. Roentgenol.* **2012**, *198*, W250–W259. [CrossRef] [PubMed]
33. Longère, B.; Chavent, M.-H.; Coisne, A.; Gkizas, C.; Pagniez, J.; Simeone, A.; Silvestri, V.; Schmidt, M.; Forman, C.; Montaigne, D.; et al. Single Breath-Hold Compressed Sensing Real-Time Cine Imaging to Assess Left Ventricular Motion in Myocardial Infarction. *Diagn. Interv. Imaging* **2020**. [CrossRef]
34. Goebel, J.; Nensa, F.; Schemuth, H.P.; Maderwald, S.; Gratz, M.; Quick, H.H.; Schlosser, T.; Nassenstein, K. Compressed Sensing Cine Imaging with High Spatial or High Temporal Resolution for Analysis of Left Ventricular Function. *J. Magn. Reson. Imaging* **2016**, *44*, 366–374. [CrossRef] [PubMed]
35. Lin, A.C.W.; Strugnell, W.; Riley, R.; Schmitt, B.; Zenge, M.; Schmidt, M.; Morris, N.R.; Hamilton-Craig, C. Higher Resolution Cine Imaging with Compressed Sensing for Accelerated Clinical Left Ventricular Evaluation. *J. Magn. Reson. Imaging* **2017**, *45*, 1693–1699. [CrossRef] [PubMed]

36. Wetzl, J.; Schmidt, M.; Pontana, F.; Longère, B.; Lugauer, F.; Maier, A.; Hornegger, J.; Forman, C. Single-Breath-Hold 3-D CINE Imaging of the Left Ventricle Using Cartesian Sampling. *MAGMA* **2017**, *31*, 19–31. [CrossRef] [PubMed]
37. Blalock, S.E.; Banka, P.; Geva, T.; Powell, A.J.; Zhou, J.; Prakash, A. Interstudy Variability in Cardiac Magnetic Resonance Imaging Measurements of Ventricular Volume, Mass, and Ejection Fraction in Repaired Tetralogy of Fallot: A Prospective Observational Study. *J. Magn. Reson. Imaging* **2013**, *38*, 829–835. [CrossRef]
38. Leiner, T.; Bogaert, J.; Friedrich, M.G.; Mohiaddin, R.; Muthurangu, V.; Myerson, S.; Powell, A.J.; Raman, S.V.; Pennell, D.J. SCMR Position Paper (2020) on Clinical Indications for Cardiovascular Magnetic Resonance. *J. Cardiovasc. Magn. Reson.* **2020**, *22*, 76. [CrossRef] [PubMed]

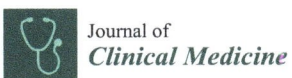

Article

60-S Retrogated Compressed Sensing 2D Cine of the Heart: Sharper Borders and Accurate Quantification

Benjamin Longère [1,*], Christos V. Gkizas [2], Augustin Coisne [1], Lucas Grenier [2], Valentina Silvestri [2], Julien Pagniez [2], Arianna Simeone [2], Justin Hennicaux [2], Michaela Schmidt [3], Christoph Forman [3], Solenn Toupin [4], David Montaigne [1] and François Pontana [1]

1. University of Lille, Inserm, CHU Lille, Institut Pasteur Lille, U1011—European Genomic Institute for Diabetes (EGID), F-59000 Lille, France; augustin.coisne@chru-lille.fr (A.C.); david.montaigne@chru-lille.fr (D.M.); francois.pontana@chru-lille.fr (F.P.)
2. CHU Lille, Department of Cardiovascular Radiology, F-59000 Lille, France; chgkizas@gmail.com (C.V.G.); lucas.grenier@chru-lille.fr (L.G.); valentina.silvestri@chru-lille.fr (V.S.); julien.pagniez@chru-lille.fr (J.P.); arianna.simeone@chru-lille.fr (A.S.); justin.hennicaux@chru-lille.fr (J.H.)
3. MR Product Innovation and Definition, Magnetic Resonance, Siemens Healthcare GmbH, 91052 Erlangen, Germany; michaela.schmidt@siemens-healthineers.com (M.S.); christoph.forman@siemens-healthineers.com (C.F.)
4. Scientific Partnerships, Siemens Healthcare France, 93200 Saint-Denis, France; solenn.toupin@siemens-healthineers.com
* Correspondence: benjamin.longere@chru-lille.fr

Citation: Longère, B.; Gkizas, C.V.; Coisne, A.; Grenier, L.; Silvestri, V.; Pagniez, J.; Simeone, A.; Hennicaux, J.; Schmidt, M.; Forman, C.; et al. 60-S Retrogated Compressed Sensing 2D Cine of the Heart: Sharper Borders and Accurate Quantification. *J. Clin. Med.* **2021**, *10*, 2417. https://doi.org/10.3390/jcm10112417

Academic Editor: Mickaël Ohana

Received: 16 March 2021
Accepted: 26 May 2021
Published: 29 May 2021

Publisher's Note: MDPI stays neutral with regard to jurisdictional claims in published maps and institutional affiliations.

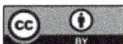

Copyright: © 2021 by the authors. Licensee MDPI, Basel, Switzerland. This article is an open access article distributed under the terms and conditions of the Creative Commons Attribution (CC BY) license (https://creativecommons.org/licenses/by/4.0/).

Abstract: Background and objective: Real-time compressed sensing cine (CS_{rt}) provides reliable quantification for both ventricles but may alter image quality. The aim of this study was to assess image quality and the accuracy of left (LV) and right ventricular (RV) volumes, ejection fraction and mass quantifications based on a retrogated segmented compressed sensing 2D cine sequence (CS_{rg}). Methods: Thirty patients were enrolled. Each patient underwent the reference retrogated segmented steady-state free precession cine sequence ($SSFP_{ref}$), the real-time CS_{rt} cine and the segmented retrogated prototype CS_{rg} sequence providing the same slices. Functional parameters quantification and image quality rating were performed on $SSFP_{ref}$ and CS_{rg} images sets. The edge sharpness, which is an estimate of the edge spread function, was assessed for the three sequences. Results: The mean scan time was: $SSFP_{ref}$ = 485.4 ± 83.3 (SD) s (95% CI: 454.3–516.5) and CS_{rg} = 58.3 ± 15.1 (SD) s (95% CI: 53.7–64.2) ($p < 0.0001$). CS_{rg} subjective image quality score (median: 4, range: 2–4) was higher than the one provided by CS_{rt} (median: 3; range: 2–4; $p = 0.0008$) and not different from $SSFP_{ref}$ overall quality score (median: 4; range: 2–4; $p = 0.31$). CS_{rg} provided similar LV and RV functional parameters to those assessed with $SSFP_{ref}$ ($p > 0.05$). Edge sharpness was significantly better with CS_{rg} (0.083 ± 0.013 (SD) pixel^{-1}, 95% CI: 0.078–0.087) than with CS_{rt} (0.070 ± 0.011 (SD) pixel^{-1}; 95% CI: 0.066–0.074; $p = 0.0004$) and not different from the reference technique (0.075 ± 0.016 (SD) pixel^{-1}; 95% CI: 0.069–0.081; $p = 0.0516$). Conclusions: CS_{rg} cine provides in one minute an accurate quantification of LV and RV functional parameters without compromising subjective and objective image quality.

Keywords: cardiac; heart; magnetic resonance; CMR; compressed sensing; fast imaging; function; retrospective; retrogating; image quality

1. Introduction

Cardiac magnetic resonance (CMR) is the reference standard method for quantification of volumes, ejection fraction (EF) and mass of left (LV) and right ventricles (RV) [1–3]. Reliable volumes assessment is required since EF has a strong prognostic value regarding clinical outcomes and survival [4–6]. However, besides steady-state free precession cine images essential for quantification, phase contrast angiography, gadolinium enhanced imaging, and additional sequences may be recommended depending on heart conditions, leading to an extended scan time, which may be difficult to handle for patients suffering from cardiac-related shortness of breath, since multiple breath-holdings are required for the acquisition [7].

To reduce acquisition time, compressed sensing (CS) has recently been applied to magnetic resonance imaging, especially CMR [8]. Based on Candès et al.'s work on signal recovery from incomplete sampling, Donoho proposed the CS acquisition [9,10]. Since the signal compression required for archiving and transfer implies the deletion of most acquired data, the principle of CS is to acquire only the pieces of information that would be preserved after this compression, sparing the time necessary for the acquisition of the data that would finally be purged during this process. Three prerequisites are mandatory for CS [11]. First, contrary to most medical images, the signal must be compressible. This means a sparsifying transform is required for most transformed coefficients to be insignificant, making the transformed image compressible. Second, the undersampling must be incoherent to provide noise-like overfolding and avoid ambiguity. Finally, non-linear iterative reconstructions enforcing image consistency with measured signal and transformed image sparsity are needed. In the case of cine imaging, the redundancy in the cardiac cycle provides a strong spatiotemporal correlation, which can be exploited for additional acceleration [12–14]. Undersampling is not only performed in plane but also in the temporal domain by using variable sampling density maps for successive frames.

The first-generation real-time CS sequence (CS_{rt}) has already been widely evaluated regarding volumes, EF and mass for both ventricles, at 1.5 and 3-Tesla [15–25]. These studies used 80 iterations to reconstruct CS_{rt} data, this setting being supposed to provide the best compromise between image quality and reconstruction time [17]. Nevertheless, computing times over one minute per slice were reported, making such a setting not compatible with clinical use [26,27]. Vermersch et al. evaluated the same sequence halving the number of iterations and demonstrated a similar agreement for the quantification of volumes, EF and mass quantification than previously reported in the literature, extending the use of CS_{rt} in clinical practice [22]. To provide an acceleration factor compatible with single-breath-hold real-time imaging, additional sensitivity encoding imaging (SENSE) and partial Fourier are implemented, the latter being a potential cause of edge sharpness impairment [28]. Another limitation is the limited temporal resolution of 49 ms which may provide variable numbers of frames per slice in the case of heart rate variability. To allow post-processing, a 25-frame per slice interpolation is performed. Besides the border blurring induced by this normalization, end-systolic volumes may be overestimated in the case of a fast heart rate [29,30].

A new generation of retrogated CS sequence (CS_{rg}) has been released. It features segmented acquisition to improve temporal resolution and partial Fourier switch-off to improve edge sharpness. The purpose of this study was to assess the image quality and the ventricular functional parameters in comparison with CS_{rt} and the reference retrogated segmented steady-state free precession cine sequence ($SSFP_{ref}$).

2. Materials and Methods

2.1. Study Population

From March to April 2019, 30 consecutive adult patients referred for rest CMR were included. Exclusion criteria were grown-up congenital heart disease work-up or follow-up, underaged patients, patients suffering from arrhythmia for whom the use of prospective ECG gating was necessary, MRI contraindications and patient refusal. Patients gave informed consent, and the protocol was approved by our Institutional Ethics Committee.

2.2. Imaging Protocol

CMR studies were performed on a 1.5-T scanner (MAGNETOM Aera, Siemens Healthcare, Erlangen, Germany). Every patient underwent three series of cine images: first the reference retrogated segmented multi-breath-hold SSFP sequence ($SSFP_{ref}$); then the CS-accelerated SSFP real-time sequence (CS_{rt}) acquired in two breath-holds, and finally the retrogated segmented SSFP prototype with CS-fashioned acceleration requiring three breath-holds (CS_{rg}). One LV 2-chamber, one RV 2-chamber, one 4-chamber slice and a LV short-axis stack covering the entire ventricles were acquired with the three above-cited sequences, providing identical slice position, thickness, and number. Imaging parameters for the three sequences are summarized in Table 1.

Table 1. Imaging parameters of the reference steady-state free precession cine, real-time compressed sensing cine and segmented retrogated compressed sensing cine.

Parameters	$SSFP_{ref}$	CS_{rt}	CS_{rg}
Repetition time—ms	3.16	2.70	2.70
Echo time—ms	1.23	1.14	1.14
Flip angle—degrees	57	60	60
Field of view—mm^2	375 × 280	360 × 270	360 × 270
Matrix—$pixels^2$	288 × 216	224 × 168	224 × 168
Spatial resolution—mm^2	1.3 × 1.3	1.6 × 1.6	1.6 × 1.6
Temporal resolution—ms	37	49	37
Slice thickness/gap—mm	8/2	8/2	8/2
Bandwidth—Hz/pixel	915	900	900
Reconstructed cardiac phases—n	-	25 [a]	-
Number of acquired cardiac phases	25 [a]	16.8 ± 3.9	25 [a]
Number of breath-holds	15.0 ± 1.2	2 [a]	3 [a]
Cycles per slice—n	8 [a]	1 [a]	2 [a]
Cycles of iterative reconstruction—n	-	40	40

Data are expressed as mean ± standard deviation in the absence of any indication. [a] Constant value. Abbreviations: $SSFP_{ref}$, reference steady-state free precession cine; CS_{rt}, real-time compressed sensing cine; CS_{rg}, segmented retrogated compressed sensing cine.

2.3. Cine Images Quality Assessment

A 3-step evaluation was performed for the three sequences.

First, a subjective overall image quality was assessed using a 4-point Likert scale (1: non diagnostic, 2: fair, 3: good, 4: excellent).

Then, acquisition quality was evaluated using a standardized score based on the "LV-function cine SSFP" section of the criteria established from the European CMR registry, evaluating the artifact detection [15] (p. 3). This score was modified, removing its four last items since their score was systematically null, accordingly to our center practice (Table 2). This score increased with acquisition impairment.

Table 2. "LV-Function cine SSFP" section of the standardized objective quality criteria score based on the European CMR registry. Adapted from [15] (p. 3).

Items	0	1	2	3	Maximum Score
1. LV coverage	Full	-	No apex	Base or ≥1 slice missing	5
2. Wrap around	No	1 slice	2 slices	≥3 slices	
3. Respiratory ghost	No	1 slice	2 slices	≥3 slices	
4. Cardiac ghost	No	1 slice	2 slices	≥3 slices	3
5. Blurring/Mistriggering	No	1 slice	2 slices	≥3 slices	
6. Metallic artifacts	No	1 slice	2 slices	≥3 slices	
7. Shimming artifacts	No	1 slice	2 slices	≥3 slices	
8. Signal loss (coil inactive)	Activated	-	Not activated		2
9. Orientation of stack	Correct	-	Incorrect	-	2
10. Slice thickness	≤10 mm	11–15 mm	-	>15 mm	3
11. Gap	≤3 mm	3–4 mm	-	>4 mm	3
12. Correct LV long axes	≥2 mm	1	-	None	3

Table 2. *Cont.*

Items	0	1	2	3	Maximum Score
Score					21
Modified score (items 1 to 8)					**10**

The four last items were nulled since acquisitions were repeated when orientation was not appropriated (item 9 = 0); all acquisitions were performed using a 8-mm thickness (item 10 score = 0) and a 2-mm gap (item 11 score = 0), horizontal and vertical long axis views were systematically acquired (item 12 score = 0). Consequently, italic criteria were not applied, and only bold criteria were used for objective quality assessment in our study, providing a maximum score of 10 points. The more artifacts there were, the higher the score was. Abbreviations: LV, left ventricle; SSFP, steady-state free precession.

Finally, the edge sharpness (ε) between myocardium and LV blood pool was measured on end-diastole 4-chamber view (Figure 1). This assessment was performed using a MATLAB (version R2015a, The MathWorks, Natick, MA, USA) homemade script. An intensity profile line was drawn perpendicularly to the mid-cavity interventricular septum border with the LV blood pool at end-diastole [31–33]. The ε value was a spatial frequency (pixel^{-1}) calculated as the inverse of the distance separating the two points corresponding to 20% and 80% of the difference between the minimum and maximum intensities along this line.

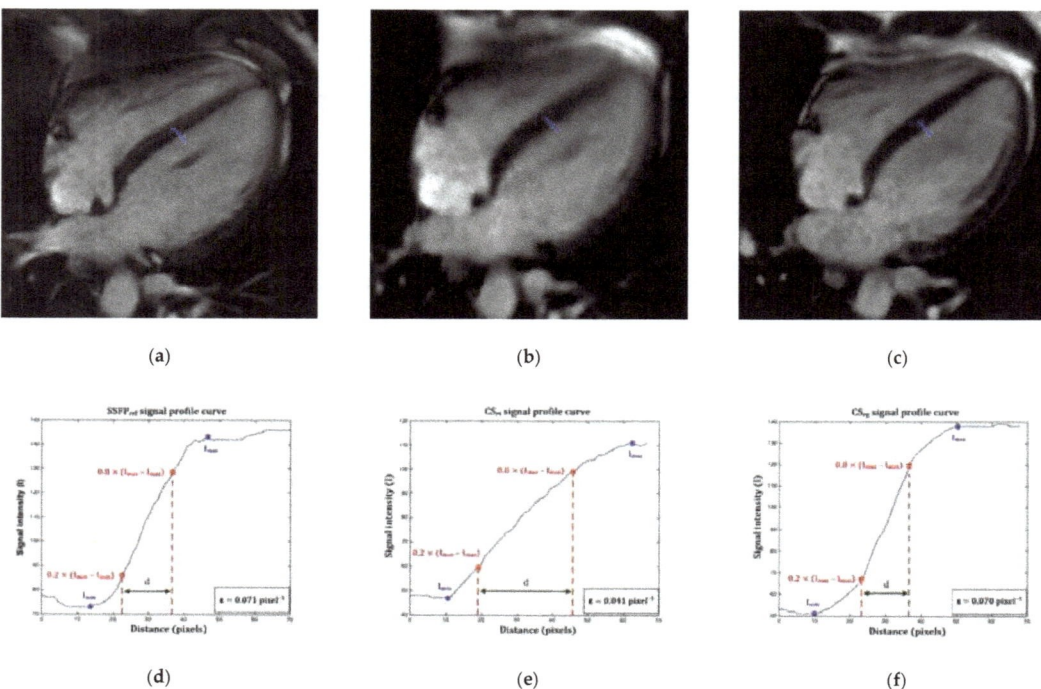

Figure 1. Edge sharpness measurement. An orthogonal profile line is drawn across the border between the interventricular myocardium and the left ventricular blood pool (blue line) on a 4-chamber view at end-diastole provided by (**a**) the reference segmented SSFP sequence, (**b**) the real-time compressed sensing sequence and (**c**) the retrogated compressed sensing prototype, providing intensity profiles (blue curves) along the line for (**d**) reference, (**e**) real-time and (**f**) prototype sequences. The edge sharpness was calculated as the inverse of the distance d (in pixels) from the positions corresponding to 20% and 80% (red stars) of the difference between the maximum and minimum signal intensities (black crosses) along the profile line and was expressed in pixel^{-1}. Abbreviations: SSFP$_{ref}$, reference steady-state free precession; CS$_{rt}$, real-time compressed sensing; CS$_{rg}$, retrogated compressed sensing; ε, edge sharpness; Ymax, maximum signal intensity; Ymin, minimum signal intensity; d, distance along the intensity (pixels).

2.4. Functional Evaluation

Assessment of end-diastolic volumes (EDV), end-systolic volumes (ESV), stroke volumes (SV) and EF were performed for both ventricles as well as LV mass (LVM). These parameters were measured on short-axis stacks with semi-automated segmentation with manual correction of the LV endocardium and epicardium while manual segmentation of the RV endocardium was necessary, using dedicated 4D analysis software (Cardiac MR analysis workflow, Syngo.via VB30A, Siemens Healthcare, Erlangen, Germany). Four-chamber, LV and RV 2-chamber slices were used to define mitral and tricuspid valve planes to ensure optimal assessment of ventricular bases.

2.5. Conditions of Image Analysis

The three datasets were independently analyzed by a 4-year experience CMR radiologist (LG). After anonymization and randomization performed for each sequence, each dataset was analyzed separately. Each analysis session, which evaluated all the images of the same sequence, was separated from the previous one by one month. A second radiologist with 11 years of experience in CMR (BL) segmented both ventricles on CS_{rg} images for interrater variability assessment.

2.6. Statistics Analysis

Categorical data were presented as numbers (percentage) and continuous variables as mean ± standard deviation (SD) (95% confidence interval (CI)) in the case of normal distribution or median (range: minimum–maximum) in other cases. Variable normality was assessed using the D'Agostino–Pearson test.

Paired Wilcoxon signed-rank test was used to compare subjective image qualities and acquisition qualities between CS_{rg} and $SSFP_{ref}$ or CS_{rt}. An analysis of variance was performed to compare edge sharpness and acquisition times of the three sequences. CS_{rg} and $SSFP_{ref}$ mean functional parameters were compared using a Student's t test, with linear regression and Bland–Altman analysis to assess the agreements between both methods. Inter and intra-observer variabilities were assessed using intra-class coefficient correlation. Significance of the test was defined by values of $p < 0.05$.

As for valvular regurgitations and WMD visualization, a receiver operating characteristic (ROC) curve was used. Statistical analysis was performed using dedicated commercially available software (MedCalc 14.8.1.0, MedCalc Software, Ostend, Belgium).

3. Results

3.1. Population Description

Demographics data are listed in Table 3. The 30 patients (22 men, 8 women; mean age: 48.0 ± 21.0 (SD) years; 95% CI: 40.2–55.9 years) were referred for: heart valve disease ($n = 7/30$; 23.3%), ischemic cardiopathy ($n = 5/30$; 16.7%); dilated cardiomyopathy ($n = 5/30$; 16.7%), myocarditis ($n = 5/30$; 16.7%), left ventricular hypertrophy ($n = 5/30$; 16.7%) and infiltrative cardiomyopathy ($n = 3/30$; 10%). All patients could fully complete CS_{rt} and CS_{rg} breath-holdings.

Table 3. Study population characteristics.

	Mean ± SD (95% CI)	Minimum Value	Maximum Value
Age—years	48.0 ± 21.0 (40.2–55.9)	18	87
Weight—kg	73.9 ± 12.1 (69.4–78.5)	53	105
Height—cm	172.5 ± 8.3 (169.4–175.6)	157	189
Body surface area—m^2	1.87 ± 0.17 (1.80–1.93)	1.55	2.22
Body mass index—kg/m^2	24.8 ± 3.6 (23.5–26.2)	19.8	33.7
Heart rate—beats per minute	73.8 ± 13.5 (68.7–78.9)	54	101

Abbreviations: SD, standard deviation; 95% CI, 95% confidence interval.

3.2. Scan Time and Image Quality

$SSFP_{ref}$ mean scan time was 485.4 ± 83.3 (SD) s (95% CI: 454.3–516.5 s) while CS_{rt} scan time was 23.9 ± 5.2 (SD) s (95% CI: 21.9–25.8 s) and CS_{rg} scan time was 58.3 ± 15.1 (SD) s (95% CI: 53.7–64.2 s) ($p < 0.0001$). Compared to $SSFP_{ref}$, the mean acceleration factor provided by CS_{rg} was 8.7 ± 2.6 (SD) (95% CI: 4.5–15.7). A mean number of 15.0 ± 1.2 (SD) slices (95% CI: 14.6–15.4 slices) was acquired with each technique. For CS_{rg} reconstruction of the full dataset, the mean time was 82.9 ± 23.4 (SD) s (95% CI: 77.4–110.1 s).

All images were rated as diagnostic. CS_{rg} subjective quality score (median: 4; range: 2–4) was higher than the one provided by CS_{rt} (median: 3; range: 2–4; $p = 0.0008$). $SSFP_{ref}$ overall quality score (median: 4; range: 2–4) was not different from CS_{rg} score ($p = 0.31$).

Regarding the acquisition quality based on the EuroCMR registry, the CS_{rg} sequence (median: 0; range: 0–3) was not different from either the $SSFP_{ref}$ acquisition (median: 0; range: 0–3; $p = 0.38$) or the CS_{rt} cine (median: 0; range: 0–3; $p = 0.83$).

The CS_{rg} demonstrated a significantly better edge sharpness than CS_{rt} (ε_{CSrg} = 0.083 ± 0.013 (SD) $pixel^{-1}$ (95% CI: 0.078–0.087 $pixel^{-1}$) versus ε_{CSrt} = 0.070 ± 0.011 (SD) $pixel^{-1}$ (95% CI: 0.066–0.074 $pixel^{-1}$); $p = 0.0004$). Moreover, no significant difference was demonstrated between CS_{rg} and $SSFP_{ref}$ ($\varepsilon_{SSFPref}$ = 0.075 ± 0.016 (SD) $pixel^{-1}$ (95% CI: 0.069–0.081 $pixel^{-1}$); $p = 0.0516$) (Figure 2; Figure 3; Video S1; Video S2 (Supplementary Materials)).

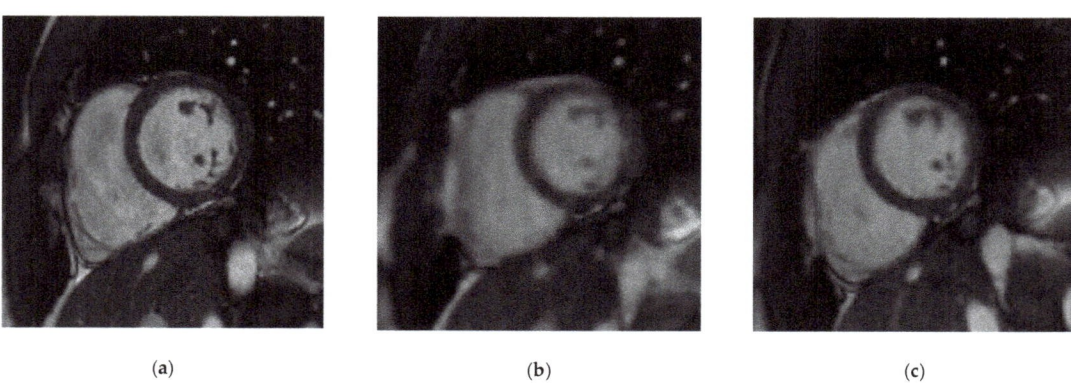

(a)   (b)   (c)

Figure 2. Midventricular short-axis cine slice acquired with the three cine sequences in a 37-year-old patient referred for myocarditis suspicion. (**a**) Reference steady-state free precession cine: Likert scale = 4/4; EuroCMR score = 0/10; $\varepsilon = 0.082$ $pixel^{-1}$; LVEF = 59%, LVEDV = 135 mL, LVM = 83 g, RVEF = 63%, RVEDV = 159 mL; (**b**) Real-time compressed sensing cine: Likert scale = 4/3; EuroCMR score = 0/10; $\varepsilon = 0.056$ $pixel^{-1}$; LVEF = 60%, LVEDV = 133 mL, LVM = 81 g, RVEF = 61%, RVEDV = 153 mL; (**c**) Retrogated compressed sensing cine: Likert scale = 4/4; EuroCMR score = 0/10; $\varepsilon = 0.081$ $pixel^{-1}$; LVEF = 58%, LVEDV = 133 mL, LVM = 86 g, RVEF = 62%, RVEDV = 164 mL. Abbreviations: ε, edge sharpness; LVEF, left ventricular ejection fraction; LVEDV, left ventricular end-diastolic volume; LVM, left ventricular myocardial mass; RVEF, right ventricular ejection fraction; RVEDV, right ventricular end-diastolic volume.

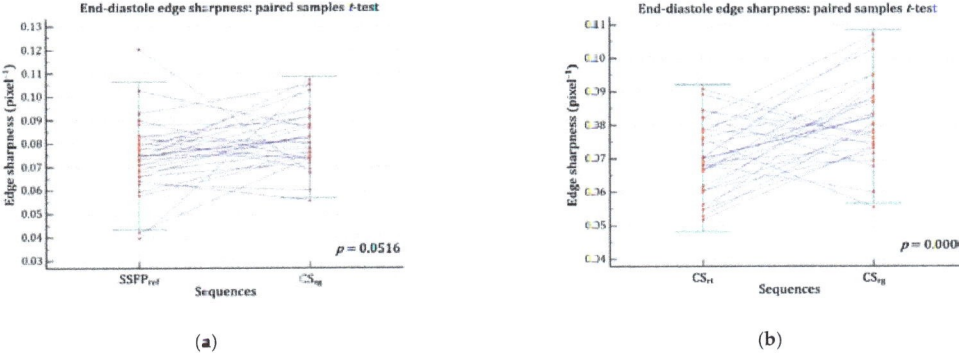

Figure 3. Edge sharpness comparison assessed at end-diastole. (**a**) There was no significant difference regarding ε between CS_{rg} and $SSFP_{ref}$ ($p = 0.0516$) (**b**) but CS_{rg} significantly improved ε while compared with CS_{rt} ($p = 0.0004$). Abbreviations: CS_{rg}, retrogated compressed sensing; CS_{rt}, real-time compressed sensing; $SSFP_{ref}$, reference steady-state free precession; ε, edge sharpness.

3.3. Volumes, Functions and Mass Quantification

Good agreements were yielded by Bland–Altman and linear regression analyses for both LV (Figure 4) and RV (Figure 5) assessments. No significant difference was demonstrated regarding LVM, LV and RV volumes (EDV, ESV, SV) and EF ($p > 0.05$) (Table 4). Intrarater variability was excellent, demonstrating intraclass correlation coefficients (ICC) greater than 0.99 for both ventricles, as were interrater variabilities for LV (ICC ≥ 0.97) and RV (ICC ≥ 0.96).

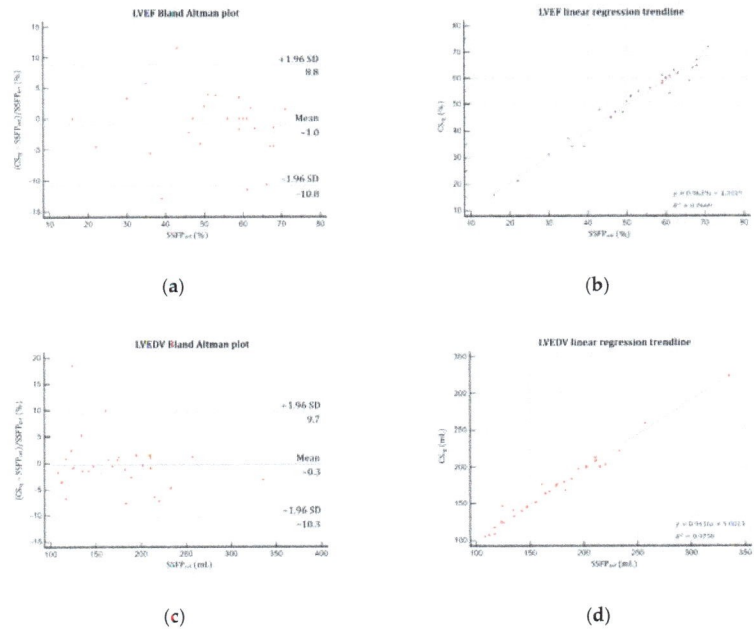

Figure 4. Cont.

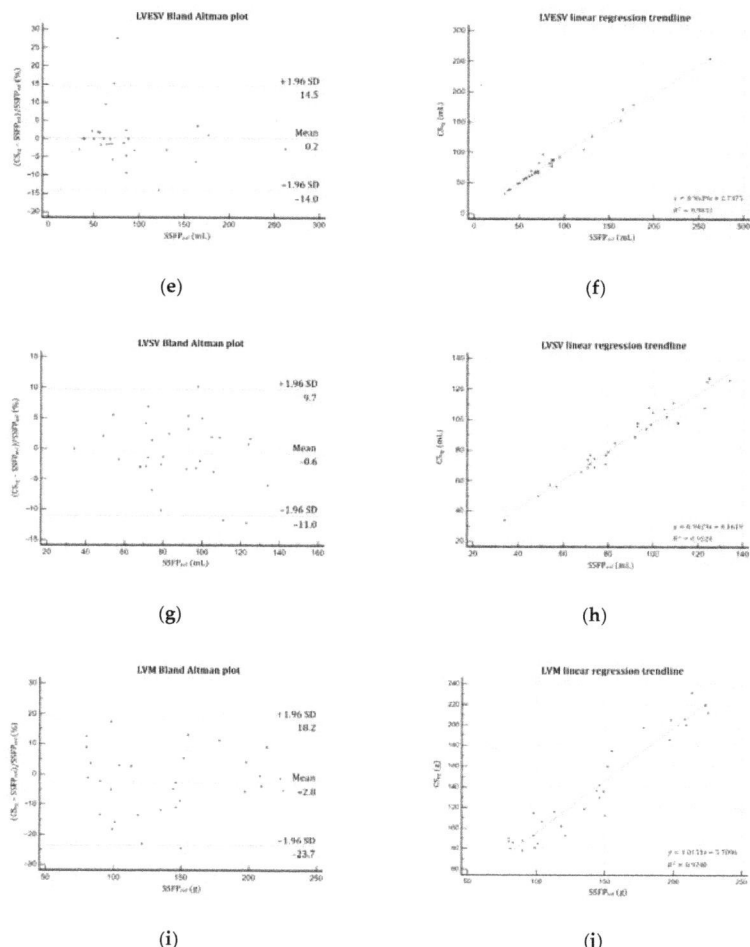

Figure 4. Bland–Altman plots and linear regression trendlines applied to left ventricular functional parameters quantifications. Left column: Bland–Altman plots for (**a**) LVEF, (**c**) LVEDV, (**e**) LVESV, (**g**) LVSV and (**i**) LVM. Solid blue lines are the mean differences between parameters measured with $SSFP_{ref}$ and CS_{rg} sequences and dashed red lines are the 95% limits of agreement. Right column: linear regression trend lines for (**b**) LVEF, (**d**) LVEDV, (**f**) LVESV, (**h**) LVSV and (**j**) LVM. Abbreviations: $SSFP_{ref}$, reference steady-state free precession; CS_{rg}, retrogated compressed sensing; SD, standard deviation; LVEF, left ventricular ejection fraction; LVEDV, left ventricular end-diastolic volume; LVESV, left ventricular end-systolic volume; LVSV, left ventricular stroke volume; LVM, left ventricular mass.

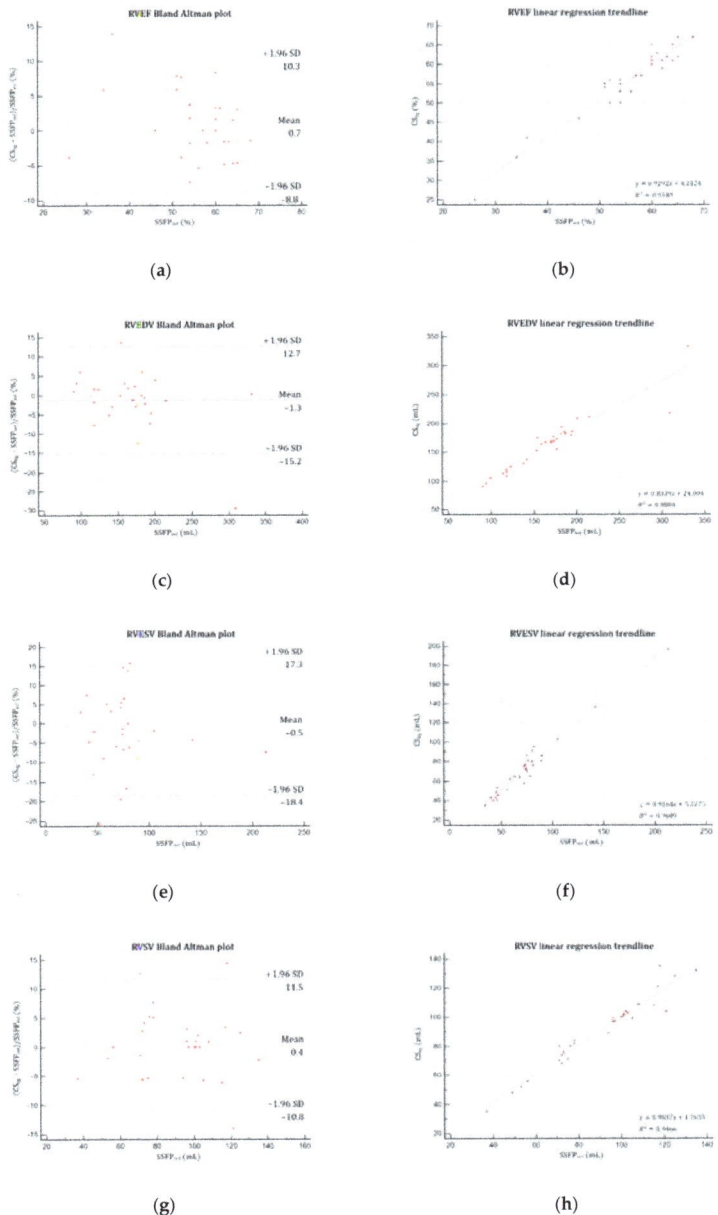

Figure 5. Bland–Altman plots and linear regression trendlines applied to right ventricular functional parameters quantifications. Left column: Bland-Altman plots for (**a**) RVEF, (**c**) RVEDV, (**e**) RVESV, and (**g**) RVSV. Solid blue lines are the mean differences between parameters measured with SSFP$_{ref}$ and CS$_{rg}$ sequences and dashed red lines are the 95% limits of agreement. Right column: linear regression trend lines for (**b**) RVEF, (**d**) RVEDV, (**f**) RVESV, and (**h**) RVSV. Abbreviations: SSFP$_{ref}$, reference steady-state free precession; CS$_{rg}$, retrogated compressed sensing; SD, standard deviation; RVEF, right ventricular ejection fraction; RVEDV, right ventricular end-diastolic volume; RVESV, right ventricular end-systolic volume; RVSV, right ventricular stroke volume.

Table 4. Functional parameters segmented on both the reference steady-state free-precession and retrogated compressed-sensing cine.

	SSFP$_{ref}$ Sequence (Mean ± SD (95% CI))	CS$_{rg}$ Sequence (Mean ± SD (95% CI))	Difference (Mean ± SD (95% CI))	Paired t Test p	ICC Inter	ICC Intra
LVEF—%	52.7 ± 14.1 (47.5–58.0)	52.1 ± 13.8 (47.0–57.3)	−0.6 ± 2.6 (−1.6 to −0.4)	0.21	0.99	0.9996
LVEDV—mL	174.1 ± 50.3 (155.3–192.9)	173.0 ± 48.0 (155.1–190.9)	−1.2 ± 8.0 (−4.2 to −1.8)	0.43	0.99	0.9994
LVESV—mL	86.8 ± 49.4 (68.4–105.2)	86.4 ± 48.0 (68.5–104.3)	−0.4 ± 6.5 (−2.8 to −2.0)	0.74	0.98	0.9906
LVSV—mL	87.5 ± 24.0 (78.6–96.5)	86.7 ± 23.2 (78.0–95.4)	−0.8 ± 5.3 (−2.8 to −1.1)	0.39	0.98	0.9932
LVM—g	139.5 ± 47.7 (121.6–157.3)	135.9 ± 50.4 (117.0–154.7)	−3.6 ± 13.9 (−8.8 to 1.6)	0.17	0.97	0.9994
RVEF—%	55.8 ± 9.7 (52.2–59.4)	56.0 ± 9.3 (52.6–59.5)	0.3 ± 2.4 (−0.7 to 1.2)	0.56	0.96	0.9965
RVEDV—mL	167.0 ± 53.6 (147.0–187.0)	163.2 ± 47.4 (145.5–180.9)	−3.8 ± 18.2 (−10.5 to 3.05)	0.27	0.98	0.9968
RVESV—mL	74.1 ± 34.3 (61.3–86.9)	73.1 ± 32.0 (61.1–85.0)	−1.0 ± 6.9 (−3.6 to 1.6)	0.45	0.96	0.9934
RVSV—mL	89.8 ± 24.3 (80.8–98.9)	90.1 ± 24.5 (81.0–99.3)	−0.3 ± 5.7 (−1.8 to 2.4)	0.77	0.97	0.9961

ICC assessed the inter and intrarater agreements for ventricular segmentations. The significance of Student's t test is defined by values of $p < 0.05$. Abbreviations: SSFP$_{ref}$, reference steady-state free-precession cine; CS$_{rg}$, retrogated compressed-sensing cine; SD, standard deviation; 95%CI, 95% confidence interval; LV, left ventricular; RV, right ventricular; EF, ejection fraction; EDV, end-diastolic volume; ESV, end-systolic volume; SV, stroke volume; LVM, left ventricular mass; ICC, intraclass correlation coefficient; Inter, interrater; Intra, intrarater.

4. Discussion

Our clinical study performed a comprehensive evaluation of a retrogated CS sequence in daily practice. Results are in line with preliminary CS$_{rg}$ tests on eight healthy volunteers reported by Forman et al., regarding LVEF, LVEDV and LVESV, which were similar to SSFP$_{ref}$ quantification [34]. However, the study population was small and LVM, RV volumes and EF were not assessed. In the present study, no significant difference was demonstrated regarding LVM, LV and RV volumes (EDV, ESV and SV) and EF.

First-generation 49-ms temporal resolution CS$_{rt}$ sequence provided LVEDV underestimation and LVM overestimation, which were clinically insignificant or smaller than intra or interrater variabilities [17,22,25,26,35]. Moreover, LVEDV underestimation was also reported with other acceleration techniques such as radial gradient-echo or k-space parallel imaging [36,37]. These differences were not depicted with CS$_{rg}$. This might be explained by the improved edge sharpness facilitating segmentation, retrospective ECG gating allowing acquisition of the last phases of the cardiac cycle and the better temporal resolution (37 ms) [38]. This observation is in line with previous studies suggesting an optimal temporal resolution for accurate steady-state free precession quantification below 45 ms [29]. Since quantification is a major CMR point of interest, the absence of significant difference regarding each LV and RV parameter seems promising for clinical implementation [1]. Moreover, the high intra and interrater reproducibility allows the use of CS$_{rg}$ for chronic status follow-up such as heart failure, anthracycline induced cardiotoxicity and other cardiomyopathies [39–41].

The overall image quality alteration using CS$_{rt}$ has already been assessed in a previous publication [22]. The higher score provided by CS$_{rg}$ confirmed the image quality improvement. Indeed, CS$_{rt}$ interpolation was responsible for smoothed images, which required physicians to get used to this rendering. The absence of difference between acquisitions qualities (EuroCMR quality score) was expected. Indeed, no difference had been demonstrated regarding the first-generation CS sequence. The evaluated prototype features partial Fourier switch-off and segmented acquisition, which were not supposed to generate more artifacts. Regarding edge sharpness, the absence of interpolation and acquisition of more data improves boarder delineation. Not only was ε_{CSrg} better than ε_{CSrg} but it was similar to $\varepsilon_{SSFPref}$. Edge sharpness was chosen as a metric for intrinsic image quality assessment due to its simple and reproducible implementation. Moreover, edge sharpness is an estimate of the edge spread function whose derivative is a line-spread function [33]. Fast Fourier transform of the latter gives the task-based modulation transfer function (MTF_{Task}); edge sharpness can be considered as a reasonable approximation of MTF_{Task}, which is widely used to evaluate the spatial frequency response of an imaging system, even using iterative reconstructions [42].

Predictably, CS_{rg} scan time was approximatively twice as long as the first-generation CS sequence since acquisitions were segmented on two heart beats in contrast to real-time imaging. However, as compared to $SSFP_{ref}$, the mean CS_{rg} scan time of about 60 s still provides an 8.7-fold acceleration factor. The study protocol divided CS_{rg} acquisition in 3 stacks to shorten breath-holdings. Nevertheless, this setting is adjustable, such as the number of heart beats required for one slice to reduce apneas or increase spatiotemporal resolution. We chose to use CS to improve scan time, with workflow fluency being a major point of concern. However, it is possible to take advantage of this acceleration to improve spatial resolution, or maybe more interestingly, temporal resolution. Indeed, in the field of feature tracking in CMR, a resolution at least over 30 frames per cycle is recommended for accurate strain assessment, which is more time-consuming when using $SSFP_{ref}$ [43]. Such settings may facilitate further feature tracking studies, though the impact of CS based reconstructions should be evaluated regarding strain analysis reliability.

The image quality improvement provided by the prototype CS_{rg} as compared to the first-generation real-time CS_{rt} should facilitate the spread of CS use in daily practice. However, the 2-shot acquisition is responsible for the loss of the real-time acquisition. Futures generations of CS cine sequences, maintaining the CS_{rt} real-time feature and the CS_{rg} image quality, should be oriented towards the application of additional motion correction algorithms to provide free-breathing acquisition with preserved image quality.

Limitations

The size of the population was limited and cannot represent the whole variety of cardiac conditions encountered in daily practice. Nevertheless, the main objective of this study was to assess the image quality recovery as compared to $SSFP_{ref}$ and CS_{rt}. To facilitate the standardized assessment of edge sharpness, we chose to exclude congenital heart disease anatomy. Among the cardiac conditions assessed by CMR, dilated cardiomyopathy is a frequent pathology, usually responsible for shortness of breath, in which the LV wall may be thinned. The decreased wall thickness may be challenging for endocardium and epicardium delineation, thus impairing LV mass assessment. The impact of LV wall thickness for this assessment, for instance in dilated cardiomyopathy, could not be evaluated because of an insufficient subgroup. Nevertheless, we assume that the edge sharpness provided by CS_{rg} should help to distinguish the endocardium from the epicardium as compared to the first-generation CS_{rt} cine that provided blurrier borders. Although a high acceleration factor was demonstrated using CS_{rg}, the improvement of CMR tolerance can only be assumed since this parameter was not evaluated. However, we suppose that the lower number of breath-holdings required by CS_{rg} should help dyspneic or claustrophobic patients undergo CMR examinations. This acceleration might be overestimated and must be interpreted cautiously since the two 1.6×1.6 mm^2 in-plane resolution CS sequences were compared with a 1.3×1.3 mm^2 in-plane resolution reference sequence. However, Miller et al. demonstrated that the maximal accuracy for functional parameters quantification using SSFP sequence was reached between 1 and 2-mm in-plane spatial resolution [29]. Even though further acquisitions could be performed during CS_{rg} reconstruction during this study ($SSFP_{ref}$ images were acquired first and available), up to 2 min were necessary for images to be reconstructed and displayed to set the next sequences orientation in case of exclusive use of CS_{rg}. Wall motion abnormalities were not evaluated, but the increased temporal resolution provided by segmented acquisition and the absence of interpolation should not impair their visualization on CS_{rg} since the first generation of compressed sensing cine was demonstrated to be reliable for this evaluation (Video S3 (Supplementary Materials)) [44]. The heart rate of the evaluated patients ranged from 54 to 101 beats per minute (R–R intervals: 594 ms to 1111 ms). Since CS_{rg} is a 2-shot sequence and its temporal resolution is constant (37 ms), the amount of data acquired during the acquisition must vary and may have an impact on the quality of the reconstructed cine images and consequently on functional assessment. The impact of heart rate on image quality was not evaluated in this study due to the limited size of the study population. Finally, only sinus rhythm patients were enrolled in this study. Even though a real-time acquisition is more robust than a segmented acquisition versus arrhythmia, the need of only two heart beats per slice should be more arrhythmia-proof than the conventional 8-heart-beat $SSFP_{ref}$. Further comparison with other acceleration techniques such as generalized autocalibrating partial parallel acquisition would be interesting since the later requires more heart beats for identical temporal and spatial resolutions [45].

5. Conclusions

CS_{rg} allows reliable quantification of LV and RV volumes, EF and mass providing similar objective and subjective image quality to $SSFP_{ref}$. Performed in clinical conditions, CS_{rg} is promising in terms of workflow improvement and image quality recovering in comparison with the first-generation real-time CS_{rt}.

Supplementary Materials: The following are available online at https://www.mdpi.com/article/10.3390/jcm10112417/s1, Video S1: Short-axis cine stacks in a 45-year-old woman referred for myocarditis follow-up; Video S2: Four-chamber cine slice in the same patient as Video S1; Video S3, short-axis mid-cavity cine slice in a 68-year-old patient referred for viability assessment after myocardial infarction, demonstrating inferolateral akinesia.

Author Contributions: B.L.: study conception and design, data collection, interpretation and analysis, drafting of the manuscript, critical revision for important intellectual content; C.V.G.: data collection and interpretation, critical revision for important intellectual content; A.C.: study conception, critical revision for important intellectual content; L.G.: data collection, interpretation and analysis, drafting of the manuscript; V.S.: data collection and interpretation, critical revision for important intellectual content; J.P.: data collection and interpretation, critical revision for important intellectual content; A.S.: data collection and interpretation, critical revision for important intellectual content; J.H.: data collection and interpretation, critical revision for important intellectual content; M.S.: study conception and design, critical revision for important intellectual content; C.F.: study conception and design, critical revision for important intellectual content; S.T.: study conception and design, critical revision for important intellectual content; D.M.: study conception, critical revision for important intellectual content; F.P.: study conception and design, data collection, interpretation and analysis, drafting of the manuscript, critical revision for important intellectual content. All authors have read and agreed to the published version of the manuscript.

Funding: This research received no external funding.

Institutional Review Board Statement: The study was approved by the research ethics committee of Lille University Hospital.

Informed Consent Statement: Informed consent was obtained from all subjects involved in the study.

Data Availability Statement: The data presented in this study are available on reasonable request from the corresponding author, subject to approval by the research ethics committee of Lille University Hospital.

Conflicts of Interest: B.L.; C.V.G; A.C.; L.G.; V.S.; J.P.; A.S.; J.H.; D.M.; F.P. have no competing interest. They are employed by an institution engaged in a contractual collaboration with Siemens Healthcare. M.S.; C.F.; S.T. are employees of Siemens Healthcare GmbH.

References

1. Pennell, D.J.; Sechtem, U.P.; Higgins, C.B.; Manning, W.J.; Pohost, G.M.; Rademakers, F.E.; van Rossum, A.C.; Shaw, L.J.; Yucel, E.K.; Society for Cardiovascular Magnetic Resonance; et al. Clinical indications for cardiovascular magnetic resonance (CMR): Consensus panel report. *Eur. Heart J.* **2004**, *25*, 1940–1965. [CrossRef]
2. Maceira, A.M.; Prasad, S.K.; Khan, M.; Pennell, D.J. Normalized left ventricular systolic and diastolic function by steady state free precession cardiovascular magnetic resonance. *J. Cardiovasc. Magn. Reson.* **2006**, *8*, 417–426. [CrossRef]
3. Maceira, A.M.; Prasad, S.K.; Khan, M.; Pennell, D.J. Reference right ventricular systolic and diastolic function normalized to age, gender and body surface area from steady-state free precession cardiovascular magnetic resonance. *Eur. Heart J.* **2006**, *27*, 2879–2888. [CrossRef]
4. Curtis, J.P.; Sokol, S.I.; Wang, Y.; Rathore, S.S.; Ko, D.T.; Jadbabaie, F.; Portnay, E.L.; Marshalko, S.J.; Radford, M.J.; Krumholz, H.M. The association of left ventricular ejection fraction, mortality, and cause of death in stable outpatients with heart failure. *J. Am. Coll. Cardiol.* **2003**, *42*, 736–742. [CrossRef]
5. Karamitsos, T.D.; Francis, J.M.; Myerson, S.; Selvanayagam, J.B.; Neubauer, S. The role of cardiovascular magnetic resonance imaging in heart failure. *J. Am. Coll. Cardiol.* **2009**, *54*, 1407–1424. [CrossRef]
6. Knauth, A.L.; Gauvreau, K.; Powell, A.J.; Landzberg, M.J.; Walsh, E.P.; Lock, J.E.; del Nido, P.J.; Geva, T. Ventricular size and function assessed by cardiac MRI predict major adverse clinical outcomes late after tetralogy of Fallot repair. *Heart Br. Card. Soc.* **2008**, *94*, 211–216. [CrossRef]
7. Kramer, C.M.; Barkhausen, J.; Flamm, S.D.; Kim, R.J.; Nagel, E. Society for Cardiovascular Magnetic Resonance Board of trustees task force on standardized protocols standardized cardiovascular magnetic resonance (CMR) protocols 2013 update. *J. Cardiovasc. Magn. Reson.* **2013**, *15*, 91. [CrossRef]
8. Vincenti, G.; Monney, P.; Chaptinel, J.; Rutz, T.; Coppo, S.; Zenge, M.O.; Schmidt, M.; Nadar, M.S.; Piccini, D.; Chèvre, P.; et al. Compressed sensing single-breath-hold CMR for fast quantification of lv function, volumes, and mass. *J. Am. Coll. Cardiol. Imaging* **2014**, *7*, 882–892. [CrossRef]
9. Candès, E.J.; Romberg, J.K.; Tao, T. Stable signal recovery from incomplete and inaccurate measurements. *Commun. Pure Appl. Math.* **2006**, *59*, 1207–1223. [CrossRef]
10. Donoho, D.L. Compressed Sensing. *IEEE Trans. Inf. Theory* **2006**, *52*, 1289–1306. [CrossRef]
11. Lustig, M.; Donoho, D.; Pauly, J.M. Sparse MRI: The application of compressed sensing for rapid MR imaging. *Magn. Reson. Med.* **2007**, *58*, 1182–1195. [CrossRef]
12. Lustig, M.; Santos, J.M.; Donoho, D.L.; Pauly, J.M. K-t SPARSE: High frame rate dynamic MRI exploiting spatio-temporal sparsity. In Proceedings of the 14th International Society for Magnetic Resonance in Medecine annual meeting, Seattle, WA, USA, 6–12 May 2006.
13. Feng, L.; Srichai, M.B.; Lim, R.P.; Harrison, A.; King, W.; Adluru, G.; Dibella, E.V.R.; Sodickson, D.K.; Otazo, R.; Kim, D. Highly Accelerated real-time cardiac cine MRI using k-t SPARSE-SENSE. *Magn. Reson. Med.* **2013**, *70*, 64–74. [CrossRef]
14. Jahnke, C.; Nagel, E.; Gebker, R.; Bornstedt, A.; Schnackenburg, B.; Kozerke, S.; Fleck, E.; Paetsch, I. Four-dimensional single breathhold magnetic resonance imaging using kt-BLAST enables reliable assessment of left- and right-ventricular volumes and mass. *J. Magn. Reson. Imaging* **2007**, *25*, 737–742. [CrossRef] [PubMed]
15. Klinke, V.; Muzzarelli, S.; Lauriers, N.; Locca, D.; Vincenti, G.; Monney, P.; Lu, C.; Nothnagel, D.; Pilz, G.; Lombardi, M.; et al. Quality assessment of cardiovascular magnetic resonance in the setting of the European CMR Registry: Description and validation of standardized criteria. *J. Cardiovasc. Magn. Reson.* **2013**, *15*, 55. [CrossRef]
16. Bogachkov, A.; Ayache, J.B.; Allen, B.D.; Murphy, I.; Carr, M.L.; Spottiswoode, B.; Schmidt, M.; Zenge, M.O.; Nadar, M.S.; Zuehlsdorff, S.; et al. Right ventricular assessment at cardiac MRI: Initial clinical experience utilizing an IS-SENSE reconstruction. *Int. J. Cardiovasc. Imaging* **2016**, *32*, 1081–1091. [CrossRef]
17. Goebel, J.; Nensa, F.; Bomas, B.; Schemuth, H.P.; Maderwald, S.; Gratz, M.; Quick, H.H.; Schlosser, T.; Nassenstein, K. Real-Time SPARSE-SENSE Cardiac Cine MR Imaging: Optimization of image reconstruction and sequence validation. *Eur. Radiol.* **2016**, *26*, 4482–4489. [CrossRef]
18. Goebel, J.; Nensa, F.; Schemuth, H.P.; Maderwald, S.; Gratz, M.; Quick, H.H.; Schlosser, T.; Nassenstein, K. Compressed sensing cine imaging with high spatial or high temporal resolution for analysis of left ventricular function. *J. Magn. Reson. Imaging* **2016**, *44*, 366–374. [CrossRef]
19. Kido, T.; Kido, T.; Nakamura, M.; Watanabe, K.; Schmidt, M.; Forman, C.; Mochizuki, T. Compressed sensing real-time cine cardiovascular magnetic resonance: Accurate assessment of left ventricular function in a single-breath-hold. *J. Cardiovasc. Magn. Reson.* **2016**, *18*, 50–60. [CrossRef]
20. Kido, T.; Kido, T.; Nakamura, M.; Watanabe, K.; Schmidt, M.; Forman, C.; Mochizuki, T. Assessment of left ventricular function and mass on free-breathing compressed sensing real-time cine imaging. *Circ. J.* **2017**, *81*, 1463–1468. [CrossRef] [PubMed]
21. Lin, A.C.W.; Strugnell, W.; Riley, R.; Schmitt, B.; Zenge, M.; Schmidt, M.; Morris, N.R.; Hamilton-Craig, C. Higher resolution cine imaging with compressed sensing for accelerated clinical left ventricular evaluation. *J. Magn. Reson. Imaging* **2017**, *45*, 1693–1699. [CrossRef]
22. Vermersch, M.; Longère, B.; Coisne, A.; Schmidt, M.; Forman, C.; Monnet, A.; Pagniez, J.; Silvestri, V.; Simeone, A.; Montaigne, D.; et al. Compressed sensing real-time cine imaging for assessment of ventricular function, volumes and mass in clinical practice. *Eur. Radiol.* **2020**, *30*, 609–619. [CrossRef]

23. Haubenreisser, H.; Henzler, T.; Budjan, J.; Sudarski, S.; Zenge, M.O.; Schmidt, M.; Nadar, M.S.; Borggrefe, M.; Schoenberg, S.O.; Papavassiliu, T. Right ventricular imaging in 25 seconds: Evaluating the use of sparse sampling cine with iterative reconstruction for volumetric analysis of the right ventricle. *Investig. Radiol.* **2016**, *51*, 379–386. [CrossRef]
24. Camargo, G.C.; Erthal, F.; Sabioni, L.; Penna, F.; Strecker, R.; Schmidt, M.; Zenge, M.O.; de Lima, R.S.L.; Gottlieb, I. Real-time cardiac magnetic resonance cine imaging with sparse sampling and iterative reconstruction for left-ventricular measures: Comparison with gold-standard segmented steady-state free precession. *Magn. Reson. Imaging* **2017**, *38*, 138–144. [CrossRef]
25. Sudarski, S.; Henzler, T.; Haubenreisser, H.; Dösch, C.; Zenge, M.O.; Schmidt, M.; Nadar, M.S.; Borggrefe, M.; Schoenberg, S.O.; Papavassiliu, T. Free-breathing sparse sampling cine mr imaging with iterative reconstruction for the assessment of left ventricular function and mass at 3.0 T. *Radiology* **2017**, *282*, 74–83. [CrossRef]
26. Vincenti, G.; Piccini, D.; Monney, P.; Chaptinel, J.; Rutz, T.; Coppo, S.; Zenge, M.O.; Schmidt, M.; Nadar, M.S.; Wang, Q.; et al. Preliminary experiences with compressed sensing multislice cine acquisitions for the assessment of left ventricular function: CV_sparse WIP. *Magn. Flash* **2013**, *55*, 26–34.
27. Goebel, J.; Nensa, F.; Schemuth, H.P.; Maderwald, S.; Quick, H.H.; Schlosser, T.; Nassenstein, K. Real-time SPARSE-SENSE cine MR imaging in atrial fibrillation: A feasibility study. *Acta Radiol.* **2017**, *58*, 922–928. [CrossRef]
28. Weiger, M.; Pruessmann, K.P.; Boesiger, P. Cardiac real-time imaging using SENSE. SENSitivity Encoding Scheme. *Magn. Reson. Med.* **2000**, *43*, 177–184. [CrossRef]
29. Miller, S.; Simonetti, O.P.; Carr, J.; Kramer, U.; Finn, J.P. MR imaging of the heart with cine true fast imaging with steady-state precession: Influence of spatial and temporal resolutions on left ventricular functional parameters. *Radiology* **2002**, *223*, 263–269. [CrossRef]
30. Roussakis, A.; Baras, P.; Seimenis, I.; Andreou, J.; Danias, P.G. Relationship of number of phases per cardiac cycle and accuracy of measurement of left ventricular volumes, ejection fraction, and mass. *J. Cardiovasc. Magn. Reson.* **2004**, *6*, 837–844. [CrossRef]
31. Wetzl, J.; Schmidt, M.; Pontana, F.; Longère, B.; Lugauer, F.; Maier, A.; Hornegger, J.; Forman, C. Single-breath-hold 3-D CINE imaging of the left ventricle using cartesian sampling. *Magma* **2017**, *31*, 19–31. [CrossRef]
32. Larson, A.C.; Kellman, P.; Arai, A.; Hirsch, G.A.; McVeigh, E.; Li, D.; Simonetti, O.P. Preliminary investigation of respiratory self-gating for free-breathing segmented cine MRI. *Magn. Reson. Med.* **2005**, *53*, 159–168. [CrossRef]
33. Richard, S.; Husarik, D.B.; Yadava, G.; Murphy, S.N.; Samei, E. Towards Task-based assessment of CT performance: System and object MTF across different reconstruction algorithms. *Med. Phys.* **2012**, *39*, 4115–4122. [CrossRef] [PubMed]
34. Forman, C.; Kroeker, R.; Schmidt, M. Accelerated 2D cine MRI featuring compressed sensing and ECG-triggered retro-gating. In Proceedings of the 25th International Society for Magnetic Resonance in Medicine annual meeting, Honolulu, HI, USA, 22–27 April 2017.
35. Semelka, R.C.; Tomei, E.; Wagner, S.; Mayo, J.; Kondo, C.; Suzuki, J.; Caputo, G.R.; Higgins, C.B. Normal left ventricular dimensions and function: Interstudy reproducibility of measurements with cine MR imaging. *Radiology* **1990**, *174*, 763–768. [CrossRef] [PubMed]
36. Voit, D.; Zhang, S.; Unterberg-Buchwald, C.; Sohns, J.M.; Lotz, J.; Frahm, J. Real-time cardiovascular magnetic resonance at 1.5 T using balanced SSFP and 40 ms resolution. *J. Cardiovasc. Magn. Reson.* **2013**, *15*, 79–86. [CrossRef] [PubMed]
37. Eberle, H.C.; Nassenstein, K.; Jensen, C.J.; Schlosser, T.; Sabin, G.V.; Naber, C.K.; Bruder, O. Rapid MR assessment of left ventricular systolic function after acute myocardial infarction using single breath-hold cine imaging with the temporal parallel acquisition technique (TPAT) and 4D guide-point modelling analysis of left ventricular function. *Eur. Radiol.* **2010**, *20*, 73–80. [CrossRef]
38. Nacif, M.S.; Zavodni, A.; Kawel, N.; Choi, E.-Y.; Lima, J.A.C.; Bluemke, D.A. Cardiac magnetic resonance imaging and its electrocardiographs (ECG): Tips and tricks. *Int. J. Cardiovasc. Imaging* **2012**, *28*, 1465–1475. [CrossRef]
39. Kotwinski, P.; Smith, G.; Sanders, J.; Cooper, J.; Kotwinski, D.; Teis, A.; Mythen, M.; Monty, G.; Jones, A.; Montgomery, H.E.; et al. CMR shows that anthracycline cardiotoxicity is common in women treated for early breast cancer and associated with undiagnosed hypertension; but cannot be reliably detected using late-gadolinium enhancement imaging. *J. Cardiovasc. Magn. Reson.* **2013**, *15*, 276. [CrossRef]
40. Patel, A.R.; Kramer, C.M. Role of cardiac magnetic resonance in the diagnosis and prognosis of nonischemic cardiomyopathy. *J. Am. Coll. Cardiol. Imaging* **2017**, *10*, 1180–1193. [CrossRef]
41. Ponikowski, P.; Voors, A.A.; Anker, S.D.; Bueno, H.; Cleland, J.G.F.; Coats, A.J.S.; Falk, V.; González-Juanatey, J.R.; Harjola, V.-P.; Jankowska, E.A.; et al. 2016 ESC Guidelines for the diagnosis and treatment of acute and chronic heart failure: The task force for the diagnosis and treatment of acute and chronic heart failure of the European Society of Cardiology (ESC). Developed with the special contribution of the Heart Failure Association (HFA) of the ESC. *Eur. J. Heart Fail.* **2016**, *18*, 891–975. [CrossRef]
42. Li, T.; Feng, H.; Xu, Z. A new analytical edge spread function fitting model for modulation transfer function measurement. *Chin. Opt. Lett.* **2011**, *9*, 031101. [CrossRef]
43. Rösner, A.; Barbosa, D.; Aarsæther, E.; Kjønås, D.; Schirmer, H.; D'hooge, J. The influence of frame rate on two-dimensional speckle-tracking strain measurements: A study on silico-simulated models and images recorded in patients. *Eur. Heart J. Cardiovasc. Imaging* **2015**, *16*, 1137–1147. [CrossRef] [PubMed]

44. Longère, B.; Chavent, M.H.; Coisne, A.; Gkizas, C.; Pagniez, J.; Simeone, A.; Silvestri, V.; Schmidt, M.; Forman, C.; Montagne, D.; et al. Single breath-hold compressed sensing real-time cine imaging to assess left ventricular motion in myocardial infraction. *Diagn. Interv. Imaging* **2020**. [CrossRef]
45. Wintersperger, B.J.; Nikolaou, K.; Dietrich, O.; Rieber, J.; Nittka, M.; Reiser, M.F.; Schoenberg, S.O. Single breath-hold real-time cine MR imaging: Improved temporal resolution using generalized autocalibrating partially parallel acquisition (GRAPPA) algorithm. *Eur. Radiol.* **2003**, *13*, 1931–1936. [CrossRef]

Article

Long-Term Imaging Follow-Up in DIPNECH: Multicenter Experience

Cécile Chung [1,2], Sébastien Bommart [3,4], Sylvain Marchand-Adam [5], Mathieu Lederlin [6], Ludovic Fournel [2,7], Marie-Christine Charpentier [8], Lionel Groussin [2,9], Marie Wislez [2,10,11], Marie-Pierre Revel [1,2] and Guillaume Chassagnon [1,2,*]

1. Department of Radiology, AP-HP. Centre, Hôpital Cochin, 75014 Paris, France; cecile.chung1@gmail.com (C.C.); marie-pierre.revel@aphp.fr (M.-P.R.)
2. Université de Paris, 85 Boulevard Saint-Germain, 75006 Paris, France; ludovic.fournel@aphp.fr (L.F.); lionel.groussin@aphp.fr (L.G.); marie.wislez@aphp.fr (M.W.)
3. Radiology Department, CHU Montpellier, Hôpital Arnaud de Villeneuve, 34090 Montpellier, France; s-bommart@chu-montpellier.fr
4. Université de Montpellier, PHYMEDEXP-INSERM U1046-CNRS UMR 9214, 34000 Montpellier, France
5. Pulmonology Department, Université François Rabelais, CHU Tours, Hôpital Bretonneau, 37000 Tours, France; s.marchandadam@univ-tours.fr
6. Department of Radiology, University of Rennes, University Hospital of Rennes, 35033 Rennes, France; mathieu.lederlin@chu-rennes.fr
7. Thoracic Surgery Department, AP-HP. Centre, Hôpital Cochin, 75014 Paris, France
8. Department of Pathology, AP-HP. Centre, Hôpital Cochin, 75014 Paris, France; marie-christine.charpentier@aphp.fr
9. Department of Endocrinology, AP-HP. Centre, Hôpital Cochin, 75014 Paris, France
10. Oncology Thoracic Unit Pulmonology Department, AP-HP. Centre, Hôpital Cochin, 75014 Paris, France
11. Université de Paris, Centre de Recherche des Cordeliers, Inserm, «Inflammation, Complement and Cancer», 75006 Paris, France
* Correspondence: guillaume.chassagnon@aphp.fr

Abstract: Diffuse pulmonary neuroendocrine cell hyperplasia (DIPNECH) is a rare pre-invasive disease whose pathophysiology remains unclear. We aimed to assess long-term evolution in imaging of DIPNECH, in order to propose follow-up recommendations. Patients with histologically confirmed DIPNECH from four centers, evaluated between 2001 and 2020, were enrolled if they had at least two available chest computed tomography (CT) exams performed at least 24 months apart. CT exams were analyzed for the presence and the evolution of DIPNECH-related CT findings. Twenty-seven patients, mostly of female gender ($n = 25/27$; 93%) were included. Longitudinal follow-up over a median 63-month duration (IQR: 31–80 months) demonstrated an increase in the size of lung nodules in 19 patients (19/27, 70%) and the occurrence of metastatic spread in three patients (3/27, 11%). The metastatic spread was limited to mediastinal lymph nodes in one patient, whereas the other two patients had both lymph node and distant metastases. The mean time interval between baseline CT scan and metastatic spread was 70 months (14, 74 and 123 months). Therefore, long-term annual imaging follow-up of DIPNECH might be appropriate to encompass the heterogeneous longitudinal behavior of this disease.

Keywords: carcinoid tumor; neoplasm metastasis; lymphatic metastasis; multidetector computed tomography; neuroendocrine cells

1. Introduction

Diffuse pulmonary neuroendocrine hyperplasia (DIPNECH) is presumed to be a rare pulmonary disorder characterized by a diffuse proliferation of pulmonary neuroendocrine cells of the airway mucosa. The proliferation may be limited to the mucosa or locally cross the basement membrane to form tumorlets or develop into carcinoid tumors [1]. Additionally, DIPNECH may result in small airway obstruction due to the combination of luminal protrusion of the neuroendocrine cells and constrictive bronchiolitis related to peribronchiolar fibrosis induced by the secretion of amines and peptides [2]. DIPNECH has been recognized as a separate entity in 1992 [3] and is distinct from reactive pulmonary neuroendocrine cells hyperplasia that can be observed in several conditions, including chronic lung disease, cigarette smoking and living at high altitude [3]. In a series of 1090 patients who received resection for primary lung carcinomas, Ruffini et al. found DIPNECH in 3 patients out of 55 with lung carcinoid tumor having a prevalence of 5.4% in this subgroup [4]. While being recognized as a pre-invasive condition for lung carcinoid tumors by the World Health Organization (WHO) [1] and being increasingly reported, DIPNECH pathophysiology remains poorly understood.

The first uncertainty regarding this disease concerns its exact definition, and to date, there is no consensus on diagnostic criteria. The WHO definition [1] is strictly based on histopathology and encompasses patients with different clinical presentations. Indeed, about one-half of patients present with pulmonary symptoms and functional impairment, whereas the other half of patients remain asymptomatic, according to the literature [5,6]. At the same time, some asymptomatic patients may present the computed tomography (CT) abnormalities usually encountered in DIPNECH (e.g., mosaic perfusion, multiple nodules and micronodules), others only present neuroendocrine hyperplasia on histopathologic examinations, and no CT anomalies. Some authors have proposed to differentiate between i/ DIPNECH syndrome in case of symptomatic diffuse pulmonary neuroendocrine cell proliferation on histology, ii/ DIPNECH in case of asymptomatic diffuse pulmonary neuroendocrine cell proliferation on histology with suggestive radiological features, and iii/ pulmonary neuroendocrine cell hyperplasia (PNECH) in case of asymptomatic diffuse pulmonary neuroendocrine cell proliferation on histology without compatible radiological findings [7]. The lack of symptoms in DIPNECH patients with signs of small airway disease on chest CT is related to the fact that small airways represent the "silent zone" of the lung where the disease might accumulate for many years with very little effect [8,9]. Chest CT and functional magnetic resonance imaging are reported to have better sensitivity than spirometry for early detection of small airway disease, as reported in cystic fibrosis children [10,11].

Uncertainties regarding DIPNECH also include the pathophysiological mechanisms and the appropriate treatment as well as long-term evolution and risk factors for poor outcome. Although DIPNECH is generally considered to be an indolent disease, some patients develop respiratory failure leading to lung transplantation [6,12] or metastatic spread [13]. Given the scarcity of longitudinal data available, there are currently no specific guidelines for DIPNECH imaging follow-up.

Therefore, the aim of this study was to assess long-term evolution in imaging in a cohort of patients with histologically proven DIPNECH, which could serve as a basis for follow-up recommendations.

2. Materials and Methods

2.1. Study Population

This retrospective multicenter study was approved by our Institutional Review Board (AAA-2019-08012) which waived the need for patients' consent.

Clinical, pathological and radiological records from 4 University hospitals were reviewed for patients with a histologically confirmed diagnosis of DIPNECH over a 19-year period, from 2001 to 2020. The diagnosis of DIPNECH encompassed DIPNECH and DIPNECH syndrome and required at least one of the following two criteria:

- either diffuse pulmonary neuroendocrine cells hyperplasia on a surgical biopsy or lung resection specimen;
- or presence of multiple pulmonary nodules on CT with one proven carcinoid lung tumor;

and:

- either symptomatic chronic obstructive airway disease in the absence of other etiology;
- or diffuse mosaic perfusion on CT in the absence of other etiology.

Exclusion criteria were the unavailability of two chest CT scans performed at least 24 months apart and the association with an unrelated active cancer.

2.2. Image Analysis

The baseline and the latest chest CT exams were retrospectively analyzed. In the case of surgical resection between these 2 CT examinations, the CT exam performed just before surgery was also analyzed. All CT exams were read in consensus by a junior radiologist (CC) and a chest radiologist (GC) with 1 and 7-year experience in chest imaging, respectively.

Baseline CT exams were analyzed for the presence of the seven different CT features reported in DIPNECH [14], namely: mosaic perfusion, pulmonary nodules, subpleural atelectasis, mucoid impactions, bronchial thickening, bronchiectasis and pulmonary cysts. Regarding the pulmonary nodules, micronodules/nodules suggestive of tumorlets (<5 mm in diameter) and nodules suggestive of carcinoid tumors ($\geq$5 mm in diameter) were counted, the size of the largest nodule was measured and the presence of calcifications, as well as central/peripheral location, were assessed. A nodule was considered to be centrally located if it was connected to a segmental or more proximal bronchus. Side-by-side comparison between baseline and follow-up CT exams was also performed to determine changes in mosaic perfusion extent, changes in size or number of pulmonary nodules and occurrence of lymphatic or metastatic spread.

2.3. Clinical Data

Patient charts were reviewed for demographic characteristics, symptoms, smoking history and pulmonary function tests (PFTs) at the time of the baseline CT scan. The diagnosis circumstances were investigated and classified into 3 categories: incidental finding, respiratory symptom or CT staging of unrelated neoplasm. The date and type of surgery, as well as histopathological results, were also retrieved.

In cases where another surgery was performed after the diagnosis of DIPNECH had already been established, the CT examination performed prior to treatment and clinical information were both reviewed.

Additionally, the latest follow-up PFTs were collected to assess the evolution of obstruction based on forced expiratory volume in 1 second (FEV_1). A decrease of at least 10% of FEV_1 absolute predicted value was considered significant.

2.4. Statistical Analysis

Statistical analysis was performed using R software (version 3.6, R Foundation, Vienna, Austria). Qualitative variables were expressed as percentages, whereas quantitative variables were expressed as the median and interquartile range (IQR). Patient characteristics and baseline CT findings were compared between patients with progressive disease requiring additional intervention and the remaining patients. Comparisons were performed using the Fisher exact test for qualitative variables and the Wilcoxon–Mann–Whitney test for quantitative variables. p values less than 0.05 were regarded as being significant.

3. Results

3.1. Patients' Characteristics at Baseline

A total of 66 patients considered to have DIPNECH were identified in the databases of four university hospitals. Of these, the 27 patients who had at least two years of CT follow-up and met the criteria for DIPNECH diagnosis were included (Figure 1, flow chart). Patients were mostly of female gender ($n = 25/27$; 93%) and had a median age of 63 years (IQR: 59–72 years; range: 42–88 years) at the time of baseline CT scan (Table 1).

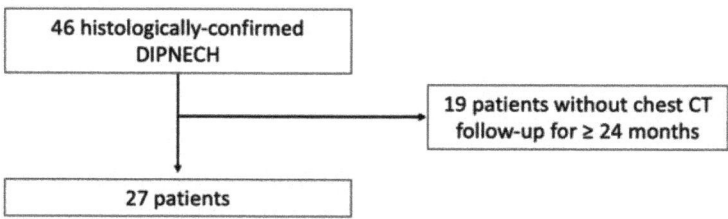

Figure 1. Flow chart.

Table 1. Patient characteristics.

	All (n = 27)	Lymphatic or Distant Metastasis (n = 3)	No Lymphatic or Distant Metastasis (n = 24)	p Value *
Female	25/27 (93)	3/3 (100%)	22/24 (92%)	1
Age * (years)	63 (59–72)	62 (61–67)	64 (59–72)	0.969
≥1 atypical carcinoid	6/27 (22%)	3/3 (100%)	3/24 (13%)	0.005
Circumstances of the Diagnosis:				0.162
Symptomatic patient	15/24 (62%)	1/3 (33%)	14/21 (67%)	
Incidental finding	5/24 (21%)	1/3 (33%)	4/21 (19%)	
Staging of unrelated neoplasm	4/24 (17%)	1/3 (33%)	3/21 (14%)	
Respiratory Symptoms:	18/22 (82%)	2/3 (67%)	16/19 (84%)	0.470
Cough	12/22 (55%)	1/3 (33%)	11/19 (58%)	0.571
Dyspnea	10/22 (45%)	0/3 (0%)	10/19 (53%)	0.221
Other respiratory symptoms	8/22 (36%)	1/3 (33%)	7/19 (37%)	1
Non-smoker	11/20 (55%)	2/2 (100%)	9/18 (50%)	0.479
Baseline PFT:				
Obstructive syndrome	9/18 (50%)	2/2 (100%)	7/16 (44%)	0.471
FEV_1 (% pred)	82 (72–89)	79 (78–80)	84 (63–90)	0.574

Note: Quantitative data are presented as median [interquartile range] and qualitative data are presented as proportion (percentage). * at time of the baseline computed tomography scan. FEV1: forced expiratory volume in 1 second, PFT: pulmonary function test.

Neuroendocrine proliferation was histologically confirmed on surgical resection specimen in 25 patients (93%), CT-guided transthoracic biopsy in one patient (4%) and ultrasound-guided biopsy of liver metastasis in one patient (4%). All patients in this series had at least one histologically confirmed lung carcinoid tumor. Atypical carcinoids were observed in six patients (n = 6/27; 22%), whereas only typical carcinoids were found in the remaining 21 patients with the limit that not all nodules were resected.

For the 24 patients for whom the information about circumstances of diagnosis was available, the majority were diagnosed because of thoracic symptoms (n = 15/24; 62%), whereas for the other nine patients, nodules were found at the initial staging of an unrelated neoplasm (n = 5/24; 21%) or incidentally (n = 4/24; 17%).

The majority of patients for whom the information was available were symptomatic (n = 18/22; 82%) with cough, dyspnea or other respiratory symptoms in 12 (n = 12/22; 55%), 10 (n = 10/22; 45%) and 8 patients (n = 8/22; 36%), respectively. Other respiratory symptoms consisted in recurrent bronchitis (n = 3/8; 38%) and unrelated obstructive sleep apnea (n = 3/8; 38%). The median delay from symptoms onset to the first CT scan was 56 months (IQR: 27–90 months; range: 0–274 months).

Most patients were non-smokers (n = 11/20; 55%). Baseline PFTs were available for 18 patients, showing an obstructive syndrome in 9 of them (n = 9/18; 50%). The median FEV_1 was 82 percent of the predicted value (IQR: 72–89%; range: 26–110%).

3.2. Imaging Findings at Baseline

All but two available baseline CT scans (25/27; 93%) were performed prior to any surgery. All patients had pulmonary nodules associated with mosaic perfusion ($n = 27/27$, 100%) (Table 2).

Table 2. Imaging findings in DIPNECH patients.

	All ($n = 27$)	Lymphatic or Distant Metastasis ($n = 3$)	No Lymphatic or Distant Metastasis ($n = 24$)	p Value *
Baseline CT Scan				
Mosaic perfusion	27/27 (100%)	3/3 (100%)	24/24 (100%)	1
Pulmonary nodules	27/27 (100%)	3/3 (100%)	24/24 (100%)	1
Pulmonary nodules < 5 mm	26/27 (96%)	3/3 (100%)	23/24 (96%)	1
≥10 nodules	20/27 (74%)	2/3 (67%)	18/24 (75%)	1
Pulmonary nodules ≥ 5 mm	24/27 (89%)	3/3 (100%)	21/24 (88%)	1
≥10 nodules	3/27 (11%)	0/3 (0%)	3/24 (13%)	1
Size of the largest nodule, mm	9 (8–13)	10 (9–11)	9 (8–17)	0.611
≥1 centrally located nodule	3/27 (11%)	0/3 (0%)	3/24 (13%)	1
≥1 calcified nodule	3/27 (11%)	0/3 (0%)	3/24 (13%)	1
Subpleural atelectasis	18/27 (67%)	2/3 (67%)	16/24 (67%)	1
Mucoid impaction	10/27 (37%)	1/3 (33%)	9/24 (38%)	1
Bronchial thickening	9/27 (33%)	1/3 (33%)	8/24 (33%)	1
Bronchiectasis	5/27 (19%)	1/3 (33%)	4/24 (17%)	0.474
Pulmonary cysts	1/27 (4%)	0/3 (0%)	1/24 (4%)	1
Lymph node enlargement	0/27 (0%)	0/3 (0%)	0/24 (0%)	1
Distant metastasis	0/27 (0%)	0/3 (0%)	0/24 (0%)	1
Interval time between baseline and follow-up chest CT (months)	63 (31–80)	101 (62–110)	62 (32–78)	0.563
Disease Evolution on CHESt CT				
Increase in mosaic perfusion	5/27 (19%)	0/3 (0%)	5/24 (21%)	1
Increase in nodule size	18/27 (67%)	3/3 (100%)	15/24 (63%)	0.529
Increase in number of nodules	17/27 (63%)	3/3 (100%)	14/24 (58%)	0.274
Lymph node enlargement	3/27 (11%)	3/3 (100%)	0/24 (0%)	<0.001
Distant metastasis	2/27 (7%)	2/3 (67%)	0/24 (0%)	0.009

Note: Quantitative data are presented as median (interquartile range) and qualitative data are presented as proportion (percentage). * at time of the baseline computed tomography scan. CT = computed tomography.

A total of 20 patients ($n = 20/27$, 74%) had 10 or more nodules measuring less than 5 mm, which are conventionally considered tumorlets, while 3 patients ($n = 3/27$, 11%) had 10 or more nodules measuring at least 5 mm, which are conventionally considered as carcinoid tumors. The remaining 7 patients had less than 10 nodules, with a median number of tumorlets and carcinoid tumors of 3 (IQR = 1–3, range: 0–7) and 2 (IQR = 1–4, range: 0–8), respectively. Only three patients had three or fewer lung nodules (tumorlets + carcinoids) on baseline chest CT, but these patients also had diffuse mosaic perfusion related to the diffuse neuroendocrine cell hyperplasia. In all three cases, the diagnosis has been confirmed by surgical biopsy showing in addition to the carcinoid tumors, multiple tumorlets (some being beyond CT resolution) and diffuse neuroendocrine cell hyperplasia. The median size of the largest nodule was 9 mm (IQR = 8–13 mm, range: 2–32 mm). Centrally located nodules, suggesting central carcinoid tumors, and calcifications were found in only three patients ($n = 3/27$, 11%).

Other features of airway involvement included band-like subpleural atelectasis in 67% of patients ($n = 18/27$), mucoid impaction in 37% ($n = 10/27$), mild bronchial thickening in 33% ($n = 9/27$) and mild cylindrical bronchiectasis in 19% ($n = 5/27$). In one patient ($n = 1/27$, 4%), the chest CT scan revealed the presence of pulmonary cysts, but pathologic evaluation of these cysts was not available. Baseline CT exams revealed no evidence of lymphatic or extrapulmonary dissemination.

3.3. Disease Evolution and Treatment

The median duration of radiological follow-up was 63 months (IQR: 31–80 months; range: 24–170 months). During this period, lung nodules increased in 19 patients ($n = 19/27$; 70%) of whom 17 (17/27, 63%) presented an increased number and 18 (18/27, 67%) a size increase, whereas nodules remained stable in the remaining eight patients ($n = 8/27$; 30%). Despite nodule increase in the majority of patients, only two patients had an additional local treatment. In the first patient, DIPNECH had been diagnosed 15 years (176 months) earlier on a surgical biopsy. The patient had Cushing's syndrome and a stable 18 mm lung nodule in the right lower lobe, which was percutaneously biopsied. The pathological study demonstrated an atypical lung carcinoid showing ACTH antibody staining and the patient was treated by stereotactic body radiotherapy. Following treatment, Cushing's disappeared but relapsed six months later. In the second patient, DIPNECH had been diagnosed 62 months earlier after wedge resections in the right upper, middle and lower lobes showed three atypical lung carcinoids along with tumorlets and pulmonary neuroendocrine cell hyperplasia. The patient was re-operated on 25 months later, for the resection of a newly appeared 15 mm nodule, which turned out to be a granuloma.

With regard to CT signs of small airway involvement, mosaic perfusion and bronchial dilatations remained stable in the majority of patients ($n = 22/27$; 81% and $n = 26/27$; 96%, respectively).

Lymph node enlargement suggestive of lymphatic spread was observed and confirmed in three patients ($n = 3/27$, 11%). All had at least one atypical lung carcinoid ($n = 3/3$; 100%).

Distant metastases occurred in two patients ($n = 2/27$, 7%), all of whom also had lymphatic dissemination. Distant and lymphatic metastases were synchronous in one patient, while in another patient, the nodal spread had preceded distant metastases by 25 months (Figure 2). Both patients developed liver metastasis and then pleural carcinomatosis. In one patient, the lung carcinoid was also metastatic to the bone.

Pathological confirmation of the metastatic stage was obtained for all patients and showed features of atypical carcinoid for all.

Therefore, three patients ($n = 3/27$, 11%) developed lymphatic spread with or without distant metastases, in a mean time interval time of 67 months following the baseline CT scan (14, 63 and 123 months). The frequency of histologically confirmed atypical carcinoids was significantly higher in patients who developed lymphatic or distant metastases (100% vs. 13%; $p = 0.005$). The other patient characteristics were not significantly different when comparing these two patient categories ($p > 0.05$) (Tables 1 and 2).

Seven patients had baseline and follow-up PFTs with a median follow-up interval of 51 months (IQR: 38–79 months; range: 24–97 months). Functional worsening was observed in four patients ($n = 4/7$; 57%) with a median FEV_1 decrease of -14.5% in absolute predicted value (-35%, -15%, -14% and -13%), whereas FEV_1 remained stable or improved in the remaining three patients (-4%, -3% and $+13\%$ in absolute predicted value).

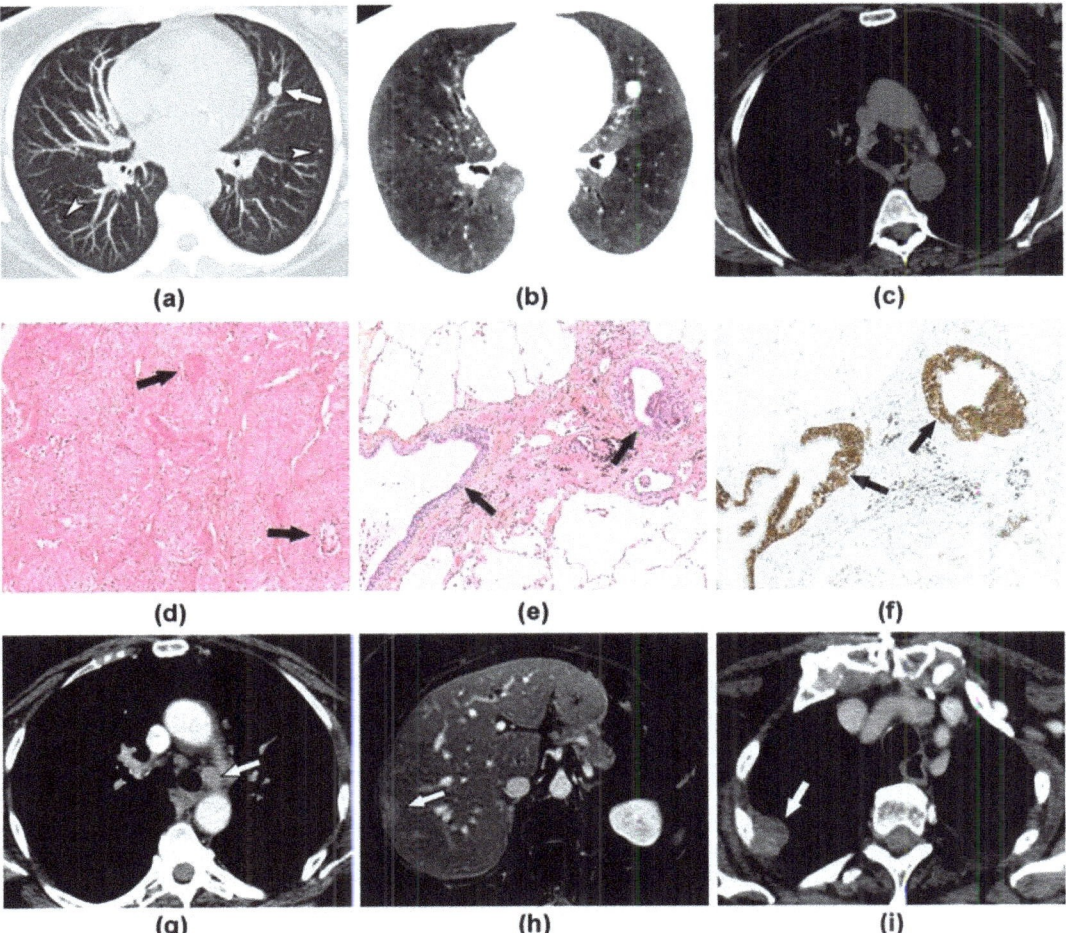

Figure 2. DIPNECH with metastatic course over an 8 year period in a 60-year-old woman. (**a**) Maximum intensity projection (MIP) reformation of baseline chest CT scan shows several nodules (arrow and arrowheads), including a 12 mm nodule in the left upper lobe (arrow). (**b**) Minimum intensity projection (MinIP) reformation reveals the characteristic association to diffuse mosaic perfusion. (**c**) There was no mediastinal lymph node enlargement. (**d**) Histopathological analysis of the 12 mm nodule shows carcinoid tumor with necrosis spots (arrows) consistent with an atypical form. (**e,f**) Analysis of distant parenchyma revealed bronchial cell proliferation (arrows) on hematoxylin and eosin stain (E), which corresponded to neuroendocrine cells hyperplasia on chromogranin A stain (F). (**g**) Five years later, contrast-enhanced CT shows the development of mediastinal lymphadenopathy leading to the new surgery. (**h**) Two years later, Gadolinium-enhanced T1 weighted axial image demonstrates liver metastasis leading to the start of chemotherapy. (**i**) Contrast-enhanced CT scan performed 6 months later shows disease progression with the occurrence of pleural metastasis (arrow). Nodal and liver metastasis were histologically confirmed and showed features of atypical lung carcinoid.

4. Discussion

In this multicenter study, we found that DIPNECH was a progressive disease in the majority of patients, over a median follow-up time of 63 months, with an increase in the size and/or number of lung nodules. Despite this evolution, the disease course remained indolent in all but three patients (11%) who developed lymphatic spread, followed by a distant metastatic spread in two patients.

To the best of our knowledge, this multicenter study is the first to focus on long-term CT follow-up in DIPNECH, and our cohort is one of the largest reported to date [5,6,15–20]. As in other reported series, we found a strong female predominance with 93% of women in our cohort compared to 79 to 100% in the literature [6,15]. Most patients (82%) were symptomatic (DIPNECH syndrome) and all had mosaic perfusion on chest CT scan, a sign of small airway disease. The median 56-month delay between the onset of symptoms and DIPNECH diagnosis is in phase with previous reports. Indeed, many patients are misdiagnosed as having late-onset asthma. However, the association of multiple lung nodules and mosaic perfusion observed in all our patients should be considered as highly suggestive of DIPNECH in middle-aged women. This association is part of the diagnostic criteria proposed by Carr et al., allowing DIPNECH to be diagnosed without histopathological confirmation [15].

Unlike some other studies, mosaic perfusion was present in all patients of our series (100% vs. 17–100%) [2,15,21]. Mosaic perfusion, which is due to vasoconstriction in areas of small airway obstruction and blood flow redistribution to normal areas [22], may be subtle on native CT images and standard lung windowing. Its detection is enhanced by the use of minimum intensity projection (minIP) reformation with narrowed window width and optimized center level settings [14,23].

Disease evolution in DIPNECH may be related to either small airway disease worsening or malignant progression. Several studies have reported an increase of pulmonary symptoms or a decline in pulmonary function in 7 to 55% of patients [5,6,15]; for some patients, functional worsening leads to end-stage respiratory failure, lung transplantation or death. Gorshtein et al. reported that 55% of patients had both functionally and radiologically progressive disease, the other remaining stable [5]. We observed increased mosaic perfusion in 19% of our patients and functional worsening in 57% of patients who had PFTs re-evaluation. By contrast, the majority of patients presented an increase in pulmonary nodules. Only two series have reported imaging follow-up data in DIPNECH patients and found a progression of lung lesions in 49 and 55% of cases but over shorter median follow durations (19.5 and 56 months vs. 63 months) [5,24]. While none of our patients were metastatic at the time of diagnosis, 11% developed a metastatic nodal or extranodal spread during the disease course. Only a few cases of metastatic spread have been reported to date in DIPNECH, the prevalence widely ranging from 0 to 27% [5,17]. The reported cases mostly consist of lymphatic spread, with only three previously reported cases of extranodal metastasis in the eye and bone [17], the adrenal gland [5] and the liver [13]. Similar to previous reports, we found metastatic disease to occur in patients with proven atypical carcinoid tumors, which was the only characteristic significantly associated with a metastatic evolution. The presence of atypical carcinoid is reported to be rare in DIPNECH, with a prevalence ranging from 0 to 27% [5,6,19]. However, in the setting of multiple bilateral nodules, not every nodule can be pathologically evaluated, and thus, the proportion of patients with atypical histology may be underestimated. Similarly, it is not possible to exclude that some typical carcinoids could metastasize, since lymphatic spread has been reported in 5% of resected typical lung carcinoid [25].

In view of the long delay, up to 123 months, between baseline CT and the occurrence of metastatic spread, long-term CT surveillance should be performed in DIPNECH. According to the current recommendations of the European Neuroendocrine Tumor Society (ENETS) on pulmonary carcinoids [26], CT scan should be performed at 3 and 6 months after treatment and then every 12 months for the first 2 years in the setting of typical pulmonary carcinoid. Then long-term annual chest X-ray and CT every 3 years are recommended. For atypical pulmonary carcinoids, closer monitoring is recommended with CT imaging 3 months post-surgery and then every 6 months for 5 years. After 5 years, an annual CT should be performed. In the setting of DIPNECH, atypical pulmonary carcinoids are presumed to be rare, and due to the diffuse nature of the disease and the advanced patient age, resection of all lesions is usually not feasible. Furthermore, an increasing number of patients are being diagnosed with DIPNECH without surgical resection, potentially leaving in place atypical carcinoids. Therefore, close long-term monitoring seems necessary in these patients. Based on our experience and previous reports, we propose contrast-enhanced CT of the chest, abdomen and pelvis at 3 months, 6 months and 12 months after baseline CT, and then long-term annual CT (Figure 3). In the case of confirmed atypical pulmonary carcinoid, the ENETS follow-up recommendations should be applied.

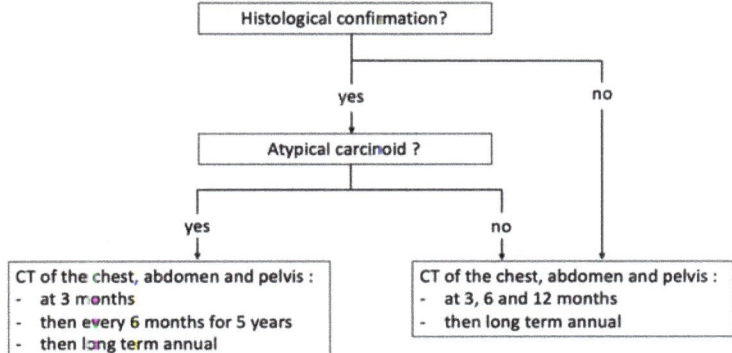

Figure 3. Proposal of follow-up recommendations for patients with DIPNECH.

Our study has several limitations; first, because of its retrospective design and the lack of available recommendations for DIPNECH follow-up, there was no standardization of imaging follow-up, and several patients could not be included due to the lack of 2-year follow-up. Others were not included because histological confirmation was lacking. We chose to propose recommendations based only on histologically proven follow-up cases. Additionally, the contribution of the 68Ga DOTATOC PET-CT scanner could not be evaluated because only a few patients underwent PET/CT in this multicenter cohort study. Finally, the limited size of our cohort made it impossible to identify significant differences other than the presence of atypical carcinoid between patients with and without metastatic spread.

5. Conclusions

In conclusion, the majority of DIPNECH patients present long-term disease progression on imaging and 11% develop metastatic spread at 63-month median follow-up. Long-term imaging follow-up is therefore required. Further prospective studies are needed to evaluate these follow-up recommendations.

Author Contributions: Conceptualization, C.C., L.F., M.-P.R. and G.C.; data curation, C.C., S.B., S.M.-A., M.L., L.F., M.-C.C., L.G. and M.W.; writing—original draft preparation, C.C. and G.C.; writing—review and editing, S.B., S.M.-A., M.L., L.F., M.-C.C., L.G., M.W. and M.-P.R.; supervision, G.C. All authors have read and agreed to the published version of the manuscript.

Funding: This research received no external funding.

Institutional Review Board Statement: The study was conducted according to the guidelines of the Declaration of Helsinki, and approved by the Institutional Review Board of Cochin Hospital (protocol code AAA-2019-08012 and approved on 16 April 2019).

Informed Consent Statement: Patient consent was waived due to the retrospective design of the study.

Data Availability Statement: Not applicable.

Conflicts of Interest: The authors declare no conflict of interest.

References

1. Travis, W.D. *WHO Classification of Tumours of Lung, Pleura, Thymus and Heart*, 4th ed.; International Agency for Research on Cancer, Ed.; World Health Organization Classification of Tumours; International Agency for Research on Cancer: Lyon, France, 2015; ISBN 978-92-832-2436-5.
2. Nassar, A.A.; Jaroszewski, D.E.; Helmers, R.A.; Colby, T.V.; Patel, B.M.; Mookadam, F. Diffuse Idiopathic Pulmonary Neuroendocrine Cell Hyperplasia: A Systematic Overview. *Am. J. Respir. Crit. Care Med.* **2011**, *184*, 8–16. [CrossRef] [PubMed]
3. Aguayo, S.M.; Miller, Y.E.; Waldron, J.A.; Bogin, R.M.; Sunday, M.E.; Staton, G.W.; Beam, W.R.; King, T.E. Brief Report: Idiopathic Diffuse Hyperplasia of Pulmonary Neuroendocrine Cells and Airways Disease. *N. Engl. J. Med.* **1992**, *327*, 1285–1288. [CrossRef] [PubMed]
4. Ruffini, E.; Bongiovanni, M.; Cavallo, A.; Filosso, P.L.; Giobbe, R.; Mancuso, M.; Molinatti, M.; Oliaro, A. The Significance of Associated Pre-Invasive Lesions in Patients Resected for Primary Lung Neoplasms. *Eur. J. Cardio Thorac. Surg. Off. J. Eur. Assoc. Cardio-Thorac. Surg.* **2004**, *26*, 165–172. [CrossRef] [PubMed]
5. Gorshtein, A.; Gross, D.J.; Barak, D.; Strenov, Y.; Refaeli, Y.; Shimon, I.; Grozinsky-Glasberg, S. Diffuse Idiopathic Pulmonary Neuroendocrine Cell Hyperplasia and the Associated Lung Neuroendocrine Tumors: Clinical Experience with a Rare Entity. *Cancer* **2012**, *118*, 612–619. [CrossRef] [PubMed]
6. Davies, S.J.; Gosney, J.R.; Hansell, D.M.; Wells, A.U.; du Bois, R.M.; Burke, M.M.; Sheppard, M.N.; Nicholson, A.G. Diffuse Idiopathic Pulmonary Neuroendocrine Cell Hyperplasia: An under-Recognised Spectrum of Disease. *Thorax* **2007**, *62*, 248–252. [CrossRef] [PubMed]
7. Rossi, G.; Cavazza, A.; Spagnolo, P.; Sverzellati, N.; Longo, L.; Jukna, A.; Montanari, G.; Carbonelli, C.; Vincenzi, G.; Bogina, G.; et al. Diffuse Idiopathic Pulmonary Neuroendocrine Cell Hyperplasia Syndrome. *Eur. Respir. J.* **2016**, *47*, 1829–1841. [CrossRef] [PubMed]
8. Hogg, J.C. Pathophysiology of Airflow Limitation in Chronic Obstructive Pulmonary Disease. *Lancet* **2004**, *364*, 709–721. [CrossRef]
9. Burgel, P.-R. The Role of Small Airways in Obstructive Airway Diseases. *Eur. Respir. Rev.* **2011**, *20*, 023–033. [CrossRef]
10. Brody, A.S. Early Morphologic Changes in the Lungs of Asymptomatic Infants and Young Children with Cystic Fibrosis. *J. Pediatr.* **2004**, *144*, 145–146. [CrossRef]
11. Mall, M.A.; Stahl, M.; Graeber, S.Y.; Sommerburg, O.; Kauczor, H.-U.; Wielpütz, M.O. Early Detection and Sensitive Monitoring of CF Lung Disease: Prospects of Improved and Safer Imaging: Early Detection and Sensitive Monitoring of CF. *Pediatr. Pulmonol.* **2016**, *51*, S49–S60. [CrossRef]
12. Walker, C.M.; Vummidi, D.; Benditt, J.O.; Godwin, J.D.; Pipavath, S. What Is DIPNECH? *Clin. Imaging* **2012**, *36*, 647–649. [CrossRef]
13. Flint, K.; Ye, C.; Henry, T.L. Diffuse Idiopathic Pulmonary Neuroendocrine Cell Hyperplasia (DIPNECH) with Liver Metastases. *BMJ Case Rep.* **2019**, *12*, e228536. [CrossRef]
14. Chassagnon, G.; Favelle, O.; Marchand-Adam, S.; De Muret, A.; Revel, M.P. DIPNECH: When to Suggest This Diagnosis on CT. *Clin. Radiol.* **2015**, *70*, 317–325. [CrossRef]
15. Carr, L.L.; Chung, J.H.; Achcar, R.D.; Lesic, Z.; Rho, J.Y.; Yagihashi, K.; Tate, R.M.; Swigris, J.J.; Kern, J.A. The Clinical Course of Diffuse Idiopathic Pulmonary Neuroendocrine Cell Hyperplasia. *Chest* **2015**, *147*, 415–422. [CrossRef]
16. Marchevsky, A.M.; Wirtschafter, E.; Walts, A.E. The Spectrum of Changes in Adults with Multifocal Pulmonary Neuroendocrine Proliferations: What Is the Minimum Set of Pathologic Criteria to Diagnose DIPNECH? *Hum. Pathol.* **2015**, *46*, 176–181. [CrossRef]
17. Aubry, M.-C.; Thomas, C.F.; Jett, J.R.; Swensen, S.J.; Myers, J.L. Significance of Multiple Carcinoid Tumors and Tumorlets in Surgical Lung Specimens. *Chest* **2007**, *131*, 1635–1643. [CrossRef]
18. Myint, Z.W.; McCormick, J.; Chauhan, A.; Behrens, E.; Anthony, L.B. Management of Diffuse Idiopathic Pulmonary Neuroendocrine Cell Hyperplasia: Review and a Single Center Experience. *Lung* **2018**, *196*, 577–581. [CrossRef]
19. Mengoli, M.C.; Rossi, G.; Cavazza, A.; Franco, R.; Marino, F.Z.; Migaldi, M.; Gnetti, L.; Silini, E.M.; Ampollini, L.; Tiseo, M.; et al. Diffuse Idiopathic Pulmonary Neuroendocrine Cell Hyperplasia (DIPNECH) Syndrome and Carcinoid Tumors with/without NECH: A Clinicopathologic, Radiologic, and Immunomolecular Comparison Study. *Am. J. Surg. Pathol.* **2018**, 1. [CrossRef]
20. Trisolini, R.; Valentini, I.; Tinelli, C.; Ferrari, M.; Guiducci, G.M.; Parri, S.N.F.; Dalpiaz, G.; Cancellieri, A. DIPNECH: Association between Histopathology and Clinical Presentation. *Lung* **2016**, *194*, 243–247. [CrossRef]
21. Lee, J.S.; Brown, K.K.; Cool, C.; Lynch, D.A. Diffuse Pulmonary Neuroendocrine Cell Hyperplasia: Radiologic and Clinical Features. *J. Comput. Assist. Tomogr.* **2002**, *26*, 180–184. [CrossRef]
22. Ryu, J.H.; Myers, J.L.; Swensen, S.J. Bronchiolar Disorders. *Am. J. Respir. Crit. Care Med.* **2003**, *168*, 1277–1292. [CrossRef] [PubMed]
23. Abbott, G.F.; Rosado-de-Christenson, M.L.; Rossi, S.E.; Suster, S. Imaging of Small Airways Disease. *J. Thorac. Imaging* **2009**, *24*, 14. [CrossRef] [PubMed]
24. Almquist, D.R.; Sonbol, M.B.; Kosiorek, H.; Halfdanarson, T.; Ross, H.J.; Jaroszewski, D. Clinical Characteristics of DIPNECH: A Retrospective Analysis. *Chest* **2020**, S0012369220321942. [CrossRef]

25. Cusumano, G.; Fournel, L.; Strano, S.; Damotte, D.; Charpentier, M.C.; Galia, A.; Terminella, A.; Nicolosi, M.; Regnard, J.F.; Alifano, M. Surgical Resection for Pulmonary Carcinoid: Long-Term Results of Multicentric Study—The Importance of Pathological N Status, More than We Thought. *Lung* **2017**, *195*, 789–798. [CrossRef] [PubMed]
26. Caplin, M.E.; Baudin, E.; Ferolla, P.; Filosso, P.; Garcia-Yuste, M.; Lim, E.; Oberg, K.; Pelosi, G.; Perren, A.; Rossi, R.E.; et al. Pulmonary Neuroendocrine (Carcinoid) Tumors: European Neuroendocrine Tumor Society Expert Consensus and Recommendations for Best Practice for Typical and Atypical Pulmonary Carcinoids. *Ann. Oncol.* **2015**, *26*, 1604–1620. [CrossRef] [PubMed]

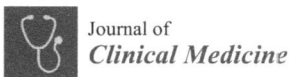

Article

Interstitial Lung Abnormalities Detected by CT in Asbestos-Exposed Subjects Are More Likely Associated to Age

François Laurent [1,2,3,*], Ilyes Benlala [1,2,3], Gael Dournes [1,2,3], Celine Gramond [4], Isabelle Thaon [5], Bénédicte Clin [6,7], Patrick Brochard [1,8], Antoine Gislard [9,10], Pascal Andujar [11,12,13,14], Soizick Chammings [14], Justine Gallet [4], Aude Lacourt [4], Fleur Delva [4], Christophe Paris [15,16], Gilbert Ferretti [17,18,19] and Jean-Claude Pairon [11,12,13,14]

1. Faculté de Médecine, Université de Bordeaux, F-33000 Bordeaux, France; ilyes.ben-lala@u-bordeaux.fr (I.B.); gael.dournes@u-bordeaux.fr (G.D.); patrick.brochard@chu-bordeaux.fr (P.B.)
2. Service d'Imagerie Médicale Radiologie Diagnostique et Thérapeutique, CHU de Bordeaux, F-33000 Bordeaux, France
3. Centre de Recherche Cardio-Thoracique de Bordeaux, INSERM U1045, Université de Bordeaux, F-33000 Bordeaux, France
4. Epicene Team, Bordeaux Population Health Research Center, INSERM UMR 1219, Université de Bordeaux, F-33000 Bordeaux, France; celine.gramond@u-bordeaux.fr (C.G.); justine.gallet@u-bordeaux.fr (J.G.); aude.lacourt@inserm.fr (A.L.); fleur.delva@chu-bordeaux.fr (F.D.)
5. Centre de Consultation de Pathologies Professionnelles, CHRU de Nancy, Université de Lorraine F-54000 Nancy, France; i.thaon@chru-nancy.fr
6. Service de Santé au Travail et Pathologie Professionnelle, CHU Caen, F-14000 Caen, France; clin-b@chu-caen.fr
7. Faculté de Médecine, Université de Caen, ANTICIPE, INSERM U1086, F-14000 Caen, France
8. Service de Médecine du Travail et de Pathologies Professionnelles, CHU de Bordeaux, F-33000 Bordeaux, France
9. Centre de Consultations de Pathologie Professionnelle, UNIROUEN, UNICAEN, ABTE, F-76000 Rouen, France; Antoine.Gislard@chu-rouen.fr
10. CHU de Rouen, Normandie Université, F-76031 Rouen, France
11. Equipe GEIC2O, INSERM U955, F-94000 Créteil, France; pascal.andujar@inserm.fr (P.A.); jc.pairon@chicreteil.fr (J.-C.P.)
12. Faculte de Santé, Université Paris-Est Créteil, F-94000 Créteil, France
13. Service de Pathologies Professionnelles et de l'Environnement, Centre Hospitalier Intercommunal Créteil, Institut Santé-Travail Paris-Est, F-94000 Créteil, France
14. Institut Interuniversitaire de Médecine du Travail de Paris-Ile de France, F-94000 Créteil, France; soizick.chammings@iimtpif.fr
15. Service de Santé au Travail et Pathologie Professionnelle, CHU Rennes, F-35000 Rennes, France; christophe.paris@inserm.fr
16. Institut de Recherche en Santé, Environnement et Travail, INSERM U1085, F-35000 Rennes, France
17. INSERM U 1209 IAB, F-38700 La Tronche, France; GFerretti@chu-grenoble.fr
18. Domaine de la Merci, Université Grenoble Alpes, F-38706 La Tronche, France
19. Service de Radiologie Diagnostique et Interventionnelle Nord, CHU Grenoble Alpes, CS 10217, F-38043 Grenoble, France
* Correspondence: francois.laurent@chu-bordeaux.fr; Tel.: +33-5-2454-9136

Citation: Laurent, F.; Benlala, I.; Dournes, G.; Gramond, C.; Thaon, I.; Clin, B.; Brochard, P.; Gislard, A.; Andujar, P.; Chammings's, S.; et al. Interstitial Lung Abnormalities Detected by CT in Asbestos-Exposed Subjects Are More Likely Associated to Age. *J. Clin. Med.* **2021**, *10*, 3130. https://doi.org/10.3390/jcm10143130

Academic Editor: Mickaël Ohana

Received: 26 May 2021
Accepted: 12 July 2021
Published: 15 July 2021

Publisher's Note: MDPI stays neutral with regard to jurisdictional claims in published maps and institutional affiliations.

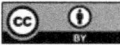

Copyright: © 2021 by the authors. Licensee MDPI, Basel, Switzerland. This article is an open access article distributed under the terms and conditions of the Creative Commons Attribution (CC BY) license (https://creativecommons.org/licenses/by/4.0/).

Abstract: Objective: the aim of this study was to evaluate the association between interstitial lung abnormalities, asbestos exposure and age in a population of retired workers previously occupationally exposed to asbestos. Methods: previously occupationally exposed former workers to asbestos eligible for a survey conducted between 2003 and 2005 in four regions of France, underwent chest CT examinations and pulmonary function testing. Industrial hygienists evaluated asbestos exposure and calculated for each subject a cumulative exposure index (CEI) to asbestos. Smoking status information was also collected in this second round of screening. Expert radiologists performed blinded independent double reading of chest CT-scans and classified interstitial lung abnormalities into: no abnormality, minor interstitial findings, interstitial findings inconsistent with UIP, possible or definite UIP. In addition, emphysema was assessed visually (none, minor: emphysema <25%, moderate: between 25 and 50% and severe: >50% of the lung). Logistic regression models adjusted for age and smoking were used to assess the relationship between interstitial lung abnormalities and occupational asbestos exposure. Results: the study population consisted of 2157 male subjects. Interstitial lung abnormalities were present in 365 (16.7%) and emphysema in 444 (20.4%). Significant positive association was found between definite or possible UIP pattern and age (OR adjusted =1.08 (95% CI: 1.02–1.13)). No association was found between interstitial abnormalities and CEI or the level of asbestos exposure. Conclusion: presence of interstitial abnormalities at HRCT was associated to aging but not to cumulative exposure index in this cohort of former workers previously occupationally exposed to asbestos.

Keywords: asbestos-exposition; HRCT; asbestosis

1. Introduction

The development and severity of asbestosis is related to intensity of exposure to asbestos and time since first exposure [1]. The surveillance of the former exposed workers is justified by financial compensations and because of the elevated risk of bronchial cancer. Therefore, and because of the long latency of asbestosis, health surveillance should be prolonged after the exposure. High resolution computed tomography (HRCT) is able to detect asbestos-induced pulmonary changes much earlier than chest x-ray and is useful for early diagnosis of asbestosis [2–4]. However, today, the prevalence of asbestosis is lower than in studies of past decades [5,6]. In addition, the pattern of asbestosis has changed and mild fibrosis has been reported [6,7]. Interstitial lung abnormalities (ILA) are defined as early interstitial changes in nondependent areas of the lung, and has been validated as evidence of subclinical interstitial lung disease (ILD) [8]. Subjects with subclinical ILD exhibit more respiratory symptoms, physiologic decline and higher mortality [9,10]. However, in a population of middle-aged to elderly subjects, ILA have been associated with a mild form of pulmonary fibrosis in smokers and non-smokers [8,10] and has been reported to increase with age [11–14]. Moreover, longitudinal studies have shown progression of imaging patterns of ILA [9] and that have been related to mortality [15]. Indeed, a recent study showed that the prevalence of HRCT patterns of usual interstitial pneumonia (UIP) and chronic interstitial pneumonia were 0.3% and 3.8%, respectively, in a smokers' cohort with 25% of progression in those who underwent a 3 year follow-up CT scan [13]. Therefore, the relationships between age, asbestos-exposure and smoking status need to be clarified.

The present study was designed to evaluate the association between interstitial abnormalities, asbestos exposure and age in a population of former workers previously occupationally exposed to asbestos. The main objective of this study was to determine whether ILA identified in a population of former asbestos-exposed workers were due to asbestosis or also to other causes of interstitial lung disease such age and/or smoking.

2. Material and Methods

2.1. Study Population

A first round of a screening program for asbestos-related diseases was held between October 2003 and December 2005 in four regions of France. Retired workers exposed to asbestos during their working life and without already compensated asbestos-related disease were eligible in this surveillance program. As previously described, volunteers were invited to participate using different ways and constituted the Asbestos-Related Diseases Cohort (ARDCO). They could beneficiate of a free medical check-up including chest CT-scan and pulmonary function tests [1,16–18]. Subjects having CT-scan sent to the regional coordinating centers constituted the Asbestos Post-Exposure Survey (APEXS) population. All male subjects of the APEXS population were included in the present study. A second round of screening was organized 5 years later and this study is based on the second round. Indeed, digitalized thin-section CT examinations of the second round of the survey showed better image quality than CT exams of the first round where a number of digitalized examinations were missing.

The study was approved by the hospital ethics committee (CPPRB Paris-Cochin n 1946 (2002), CPP Ile De France III n 1946/11/02-02 (2010)). All participants received information about the study and gave their written informed consent.

2.2. Asbestos Exposure and Smoking Status

All subjects completed a standardized questionnaire, having different parts: all successive jobs (date of beginning and end, location of the employer, main activity of the firm, precise job of the subject), indication of having ever worked in a list of specific jobs (known for high probability of exposure to asbestos) in the construction industry with indication of date of beginning and end of these jobs. 9 specific questions on tasks entailing exposure to asbestos with indication of date of beginning and end of each task; and finally free text to invite the subject to add any precision he would prefer to add to his previous answers. Therefore, industrial hygienists could evaluate asbestos exposure based on of the complete working life history of each subject. For each job considered exposed to asbestos, the duration (expressed in years) and dates of exposure were determined. The maximum level of exposure was defined as the highest exposure occurring during the entire work history. The following weighting factors were decided for the intensity level of exposure, based on the knowledge of the different situations of exposure: low (passive exposure): 0.01; low intermediate: 0.1; high intermediate: 1; high: 10. A cumulative exposure index (CEI) to asbestos was then calculated for each subject over his working life. It was calculated by summing the exposures calculated for each exposed job (duration x weighting factor). There were no atmospheric measurements in this cohort, and detailed information on the frequency of exposure (percentage of the working time) was frequently lacking. Therefore, the CEI was expressed in exposure units x years rather than fibers/mL x years. The elapsed time between the beginning of the first job considered to be exposed to asbestos and the date of CT scan was calculated as the time since first exposure (TSFE) [16–18].

The questionnaire also collected information on smoking status, allowing classification of subjects into three categories: current smokers, ex-smokers (those who had stopped smoking for at least one year) and never-smokers (having smoked less than 100 cigarettes over the working life).

2.3. CT Scanning

A specific protocol was established by a group of chest radiologists as previously described [1]. Four experts trained in the interpretation of asbestos-related CT abnormalities performed a double-blinded independent evaluation of all CT examinations. Triple evaluation was performed in the case of disagreement between the first two readings. These evaluations were performed in a blinded fashion to the subject's cumulative exposure to asbestos and to the report of the initial reading made by the radiologists who performed the CT examination. Interstitial or pleural abnormalities were registered using a standardized form according to the Fleischner Society glossary of terms [19].

The reader was asked to classify the patient into one of four categories for parenchymal findings: no abnormality, minor interstitial findings, interstitial findings inconsistent with UIP, possible or definite UIP. The second category was based on the description of abnormal interstitial findings in aging people [11] and the 2 last categories based on the consensus ATS/ERS criteria for the diagnosis of idiopathic pulmonary fibrosis (IPF) [20]. Severity of emphysema was assessed visually on a 4-level scale (none, minor: emphysema occupying less than 25%, moderate: between 25 and 50% and severe: more than 50% of the whole pulmonary volume).

2.4. Statistical Analysis

The relationship between interstitial lung abnormalities and occupational asbestos exposure was estimated using logistic regression models adjusted for age and smoking (never smokers, ex-smokers and current smokers). Occupational asbestos exposure was characterized by the CEI, time since first exposure and the maximum level of exposure.

Linearity of quantitative variables was examined using fractional polynomial [21]. Supplementary analyses were conducted to study the association between severity emphysema at CT and occupational asbestos exposure using the same analysis strategy as described above. Statistical analyses were carried out using SAS software version 9.4 (SAS Institute, Inc, Cary, NC, USA) and R software version 3.4.2.

3. Results

3.1. Subjects' Demographic Data, Smoking Data, Asbestos Exposure and Frequency of Interstitial Abnormalities at CT

At the second round of the screening program proposed to the APEXS population, 2268 subjects have been explored by CT with a double readings and triple reading if discordances. After exclusion of 92 women and 19 subjects with missing data for smoking status, the study population consisted of 2157 male subjects (Figure 1). Pleural plaques were present in 559 (25.7%) subjects, interstitial abnormalities in 365 (16.7%), emphysema in 444 (20.4%) (Table 1).

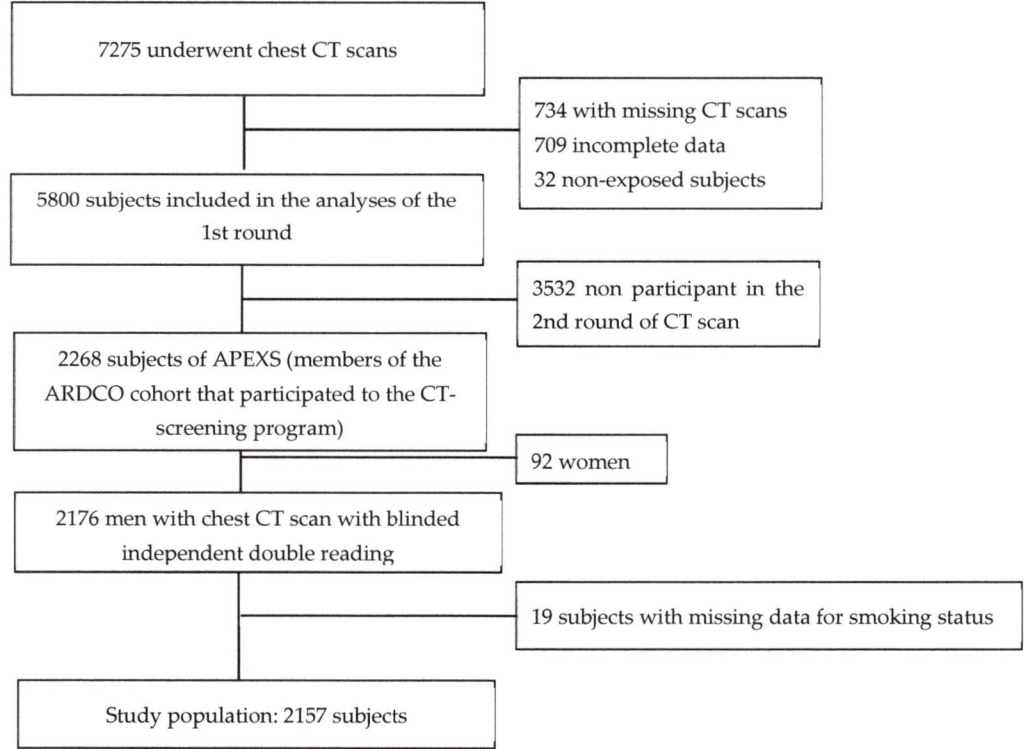

Figure 1. Study Flow-Chart. APEXS: Asbestos Post-Exposure Survey; ARDCO: Asbestos-Related Diseases Cohort; CT = computed tomography.

Table 1. Frequency of pleural plaques, interstitial abnormalities and emphysema as detected at CT (*n* = 2157).

	n	%
Pleural plaques		
No	1604	74.4
Yes	553	25.6

Table 1. Cont.

	n	%
Interstitial abnormalities		
Absent or gravity-dependent opacities	1794	83.2
Minor interstitial abnormalities	226	10.5
Interstitial pattern inconsistent with UIP	82	3.8
UIP pattern or possible UIP pattern	55	2.5
Emphysema		
None	1716	79.5
Minor (less than 25% of lung volume)	281	13.0
Moderate (25% to 50%)	104	4.8
Severe (more than 50% of lung volume)	56	2.6

UIP: usual interstitial pneumonia.

3.2. Association between Possible and Definite CT Patterns of UIP and Age, Smoking Status and the Level of Exposure to Asbestos

The frequency of interstitial findings according to demographic data, smoking status and asbestos exposure is shown Table 2.

A significant positive association was found between UIP pattern or possible UIP pattern and age (OR $_{crude}$ = 1.08 (95% CI: 1.03–1.13) and OR $_{adjusted}$ = 1.08 (95% CI 1.02–1.13)) for each additional year (Table 3).

In addition, UIP pattern or possible UIP pattern were significantly associated to smoking status (OR $_{crude}$ for ex-smoker = 2.13 (95% CI: 1.03–4.39)) (Table 3).

Table 2. Frequency of interstitial abnormalities detected at CT according to demographic characteristics, smoking status and asbestos exposure data.

	Absent or Gravity-Dependent Opacities		Minor Interstitial Abnormalities		Interstitial Abnormalities Inconsistent with UIP		UIP Pattern or Possible UIP Pattern	
	n	%	n	%	n	%	n	%
Age (years)								
Mean (SD)	69.4 (5.4)		71.5 (5.0)		72.4 (6.7)		72.3 (4.9)	
Smoking status								
Non-smoker	519	28.9	69	30.5	22	26.8	9	16.4
Ex-smoker	1163	64.8	150	66.4	56	68.3	43	78.2
Smoker	112	6.2	7	3.1	4	4.9	3	5.5
Maximum Level of Exposure Based on Labor History								
Low + Low intermediate	518	28.9	50	22.1	20	24.4	17	30.9
High intermediate	843	47.0	127	56.2	43	52.4	17	30.9
High	433	24.1	49	21.7	19	23.2	21	38.2
CEI to Asbestos (Unit of Exposure x Years)								
(0–3.3)	352	19.6	37	16.4	12	14.6	11	20.0
(3.3–13.6)	353	19.7	35	15.5	12	14.6	10	18.2
(13.6–32)	362	20.2	53	23.5	22	26.8	9	16.4
(32–64)	373	20.8	59	26.1	20	24.4	12	21.8
(64 and more)	354	19.7	42	18.6	16	19.5	13	23.6
Mean (SD)	60.6 (99.1)		58.0 (90.7)		63.0 (97.3)		72.4 (110.4)	
Time Since First Exposure (Years)								
<40	120	6.7	5	2.2	5	6.1	3	5.5
(40–50)	623	34.7	59	26.1	17	20.7	14	25.5
>50	1051	58.6	162	71.7	60	73.2	38	69.1
Mean (SD)	50.2 (7.0)		52.7 (6.14)		52.6 (7.2)		52.4 (7.34)	
Duration of Exposure to Asbestos (years)								
<10	84	4.7	7	3.1	2	2.4	4	7.3
(10–20)	161	9.0	15	6.6	6	7.3	5	9.1
(20–30)	298	16.6	39	17.3	7	8.5	7	12.7
(30–40)	829	46.2	107	47.3	46	56.1	25	45.5
>40	422	23.5	58	25.7	21	25.6	14	25.5
Mean (SD)	31.9 (10.1)		32.9 (9.1)		33.9 (8.8)		31.7 (11.5)	

CEI: cumulative exposure index to asbestos.

Table 3. Association between the possible or definite UIP pattern at CT, asbestos exposure and age unadjusted and adjusted on age, occupational asbestos exposure and smoking status.

	Univariate Model OR (IC95%)	Multivariate Models OR (IC95%)	OR (IC95%)
Duration of exposure (year)	0.99 (0.97–1.02)	-	-
Time since the first exposure (year)	**1.04 (1.00–1.08)**	1.00 (0.96–1.04)	1.00 (0.96–1.04)
Maximum level of exposure			
Low + Low intermediate (n = 605)	1		1
Intermediate high (n = 1030)	0.58 (0.29–1.15)	-	0.58 (0.29–1.15)
High (n = 522)	1.45 (0.76–2.78)		1.39 (0.71–2.69)
CEI to asbestos (100 units of exposure x years)	1.12 (0.88–1.42)	1.09 (0.85–1.40)	-
Age at the time of CT examination (year)	**1.08 (1.03–1.13)**	**1.08 (1.03–1.13)**	**1.08 (1.03–1.13)**
Smoking status			
Non-smoker (n = 619)	1	1	1
Ex-smoker (n = 1412)	**2.13 (1.03–4.39)**	2.03 (0.98–4.21)	1.92 (0.92–4.00)
Smoker (n = 126)	1.65 (0.44–6.19)	1.97 (0.52–7.47)	1.86 (0.49–7.06)

CEI: cumulative exposure index to asbestos. Bold values indicate statistical significance.

There was no significant association between interstitial lung abnormalities and asbestos exposure assessed either by CEI or by maximum level of exposure (Table 3). We have also combined the two intermediate categories of maximum level of exposure (intermediate low + intermediate high) and the results were not significant (data not shown).

When patients with either definite UIP pattern or possible UIP pattern and inconsistent with UIP pattern were grouped, this association with age remained significant (OR $_{crude}$ = 1.09 (95% CI: 1.06–1.12) and OR $_{adjusted}$ = 1.09 (1.05–1.13)) (Supplementary Table S1). On the other hand, the association with asbestos exposure remained non-significant (Supplementary Table S1).

3.3. Association between CT Severity of Emphysema and Age, Smoking Status and the Level of Exposure to Asbestos

The frequency of emphysema findings according to demographic data, smoking status and asbestos exposure is shown in Table 4. No association was found between emphysema and CEI to asbestos, but an association was observed with the maximum level of exposure to asbestos (OR $_{crude}$ = 2.05 (95% CI: 1.06–3.99) and OR $_{adjusted}$ = 2.27 (95% CI: 1.08–4.80) for subjects with "high-level" of asbestos exposure). As expected, a significant association was found between emphysema and smoking status (Supplementary Table S2).

Table 4. Frequency of emphysema at CT according to age, smoking status and asbestos exposure data.

	No Emphysema		Minimal Emphysema		Moderate Emphysema (25% to 50%)		Severe Emphysema (More than 50%)	
	n	%	n	%	n	%	n	%
Age (years)								
Mean (SD)	69.8 (5.4)		70.1 (5.6)		69.2 (5.1)		69.7 (6.2)	
Smoking Status								
Non smoker	558	32.5	51	18.1	6	5.8	4	7.1
Ex-smoker	1080	62.9	208	74.0	82	78.8	42	75.0
Smoker	78	4.5	22	7.8	16	15.4	10	17.9
Maximum Level of Exposure								
Low + Low intermediate	500	29.1	72	25.6	25	24	8	14.3
High intermediate	816	47.6	135	48.0	55	52.9	24	42.9
High	400	23.3	74	26.3	24	23.1	24	42.9
CEI to Asbestos (Unit of Exposure x Years)								
(0–3.3)	334	19.5	54	19.2	16	15.4	8	14.3
(3.3–13.6)	337	19.6	43	15.3	22	21.2	8	14.3
(13.6–32)	341	19.9	61	21.7	26	25.0	18	32.1
(32–64)	373	21.7	64	22.8	21	20.2	6	10.7

Table 4. Cont.

	No Emphysema		Minimal Emphysema		Moderate Emphysema (25% to 50%)		Severe Emphysema (More than 50%)	
	n	%	n	%	n	%	n	%
(64 and more)	331	19.3	59	21.0	19	18.3	16	28.6
Mean (SD)	60.0 (98.3)		64.2 (100.5)		60.0 (98.7)		68.1 (94.5)	
Time Since First Exposure (Years)								
<40	104	6.1	18	6.4	4	3.8	7	12.5
(40–50)	573	33.4	85	30.2	36	34.6	19	33.9
>50	1039	60.5	178	63.3	64	61.5	30	53.6
Mean (SD)	50.6 (7.1)		51.0 (6.6)		50.8 (6.5)		49.8 (7.9)	
Duration (Years)								
<10	75	4.4	11	3.9	7	6.7	4	7.1
(10–20)	139	8.1	29	10.3	10	9.6	9	16.1
(20–30)	278	16.2	43	15.3	20	19.2	10	17.9
(30–40)	814	47.4	135	48.0	38	36.5	20	35.7
>40	410	23.9	63	22.4	29	27.9	13	23.2
Mean (SD)	32.2 (9.9)		32.0 (9.6)		31.1 (10.9)		29.2 (11.3)	

CEI: cumulative exposure index to asbestos.

4. Discussion

This study has shown the association between interstitial abnormalities and age after adjustment on smoking status and asbestos exposure in a population of retired workers previously occupationally exposed to asbestos. This result is consistent with the CT lung cancer screening study by Vehmas et al. [22] among asbestos-exposed workers, where a positive correlation was found between interstitial lung abnormalities at CT and aging after adjustment to smoking status, asbestos exposure and body mass index.

The strengths of our study are the large number of subjects, individual estimation of cumulative occupational exposure to asbestos, HRCT acquisition and accurate analysis of CT by experts and categorization of interstitial abnormalities according to the ATS/ERS consensus criteria [20]. However, our analysis predates international consensus guideline for the diagnosis of IPF [23]. Nevertheless, definitions of UIP patterns are quite similar.

In a population of middle-aged to elderly subjects without occupational exposure, the presence of discrete lung parenchymal abnormalities has been reported to increase with age [11,24]. Jin et al. reported a positive association of fibrotic ILA at HRCT and age [25]. In this case, 60% of healthy subjects aged 75 or older have shown a basal reticular pattern whereas in those younger than 55 years old, no interstitial abnormalities have been reported [11]. This may be due to elastic degradation with aging, which leads to alveolar collapse or to mild interstitial fibrosis. In addition, interlobular septae thickening has been found more commonly in older subjects. However, subpleural lines may disappear at imaging in prone position in some healthy individuals. A study by Gamsu et al. [3] showed that CT findings of asbestosis are neither perfectly sensitive nor specific for asbestosis. In another study by Copley et al., the results of CT evaluation of 74 patients with asbestosis were compared to those of 212 patients with idiopathic pulmonary fibrosis showing that HRCT patterns of asbestosis are closely akin to the UIP pattern [26]. HRCT is today an essential component of the diagnostic pathway in interstitial lung disease. In order to clarify the management of patient with IPF, ATS/ERS guidelines have been published to assess the probability of the disease according to patterns [20].

Asbestosis, however, cannot be distinguished by HRCT from a possible or definite UIP pattern [26]. The first round of screening of this cohort has been reported [1] and conversely to the agreement between trained expert readers for the detection of pleural plaques that was good to excellent, the agreement between trained expert readers for the detection of interstitial abnormalities has been reported to be fair to good [27]. In an attempt to circumvent the subjects with possible mild or moderate asbestosis, we separated those subjects from those with an interstitial pattern inconsistent with UIP, using the criteria defined by ATS/ERS consensus paper [20]. Patterns with upper lobe or middle lung interstitial abnormalities predominance, predominance of ground-glass opacities, nodular pattern, peribronchial pattern, cysts and/or air trapping or mosaic attenuation in three or more lobes were classified globally in the group inconsistent with UIP pattern [20]. Interestingly in these subjects, interstitial abnormalities were not associated with exposure but with age, even when adjusted on smoking status. However, the non-association between interstitial lung abnormalities and asbestos exposure evaluated using time related markers (i.e., duration of exposure and time since the first exposure) could be related to an over-adjustment with age. Nevertheless, the association between interstitial abnormalities with typical or atypical UIP pattern and age has been reported [15,25,26]. Therefore, these subjects may have a preclinical interstitial lung disease rather than asbestosis.

In our study, the association of UIP or possible UIP pattern at HRCT and smoking in univariate analysis is in line with literature showing that tobacco consumption is a risk factor for development of fibrotic lung abnormalities [28]. This finding was not significant in current smokers which could be explained by the low number of current smokers at the time of the study (n = 126). In the study by Jin et al., the association between ILA at HRCT and smoking status was found not significant [25]. However, fibrotic ILAs were differentiated into subtypes (i.e., patients with ground glass opacities: n = 12, reticulations: n = 9 and honeycombing: n = 9) which decreased the strength of the statistical analysis. Nonetheless, in the multivariate model when adjusted for occupational asbestos exposure and age, association with cigarette smoking was found not significant.

The relationships between emphysema and asbestos exposure remain unclear. A positive association was found between emphysema and the maximum level of asbestos exposure but not with the CEI to asbestos. Indeed, CEI is considered as a more precise parameter taking into account the total asbestos exposure along the working carrier, which could be more relevant than the maximum level of exposure that could possibly intermingles other associated exposures. In addition, in a population of heavily exposed people to asbestos, Huuskonen et al. [29] have reported an association between emphysema findings and asbestos exposure, after adjustment for age and smoking. They have differentiated, however, emphysema subtypes and used a more detailed score than we did. The causative role of asbestos on emphysema remains to be determined.

Our study had several limitations. Exclusion of already compensated subjects before the first round of this survey may introduce some selection bias. Moreover, this was a voluntary based participation survey thus, motivations of subjects to not participate in the second round were unknown CT images evaluated in this study were acquired at the second round of screening, where all the examinations were stored on digital support for expert analysis in contrast with first round screening examinations that were already reported [1]. Regarding the asbestos exposure evaluation, no atmospheric measurements was performed in this cohort and detailed information on the frequency of exposure was lacking. Therefore, the CEI was expressed in exposure units x years rather than in fibers/mL x years. However, the semi-quantitative analysis of exposure with ordinal classes allowed us to evaluate the association between increasing exposure levels and interstitial lung abnormalities. The low prevalence of asbestosis in this population is in agreement with recent data in the asbestosis epidemiology [5]. However, since this cohort is based on voluntary participation and subjects who have been already compensated for asbestos-related occupational disease before entering the survey were not included, it is likely than a substantial fraction of subjects with overt asbestosis were not included in the study. There was no histological proof of asbestosis in our population. However, the diagnosis is currently made on the basis of HRCT and an appropriate history of asbestos exposure. Indeed, as a consensus, no surgical lung biopsy is needed in these patients. In addition, we have no control group, but ethical considerations prevent the use of radiation exposure due to CT in non-asbestos-exposed subjects.

We have reported that the presence of interstitial abnormalities at HRCT was not associated to the level of exposure in a population of asbestos-exposed subjects, but to aging. This should raise the issue of ILA as an early stage of IPF with a need of an adequate surveillance.

Supplementary Materials: The following are available online at https://www.mdpi.com/article/10.3390/jcm10143130/s1. Table S1: Association between the presence of UIP pattern (definite. possible UIP pattern) and interstitial pattern inconsistent with UIP pattern at CT and asbestos exposure, age, and smoking status. Table S2: Association between emphysema at CT and asbestos exposure. Table S3: Most represented occupations (ISCO 68) in the general population (n = 2157) and according interstitial abnormalities detected at CT. Table S4: Most represented industries (ISIC Rev 2) in all subjects and according interstitial abnormalities detected at CT.

Author Contributions: Conceptualization, F.L., C.P., G.F. and J.-C.P.; methodology, C.G., A.L., J.G., J.-C.P.; validation, F.L., I.B., G.D. and J.-C.P.; formal analysis, F.L., I.B., G.D., C.G., J.G., A.L. and J.-C.P.; investigation, F.L., I.B., G.D., I.T., B.C., P.B., A.G., P.A., S.C., C.P., G.F. and J.-C.P.; resources, F.L., I.B., G.D., I.T., B.C., P.B., A.G., P.A., S.C., F.D., C.P., G.F. and J.-C.P.; data curation, C.G., J.G., A.L.; writing—original draft preparation, F.L. and I.B.; writing—review and editing, F.L., I.B., G.D., C.G., I.T., B.C., P.B., A.G., P.A., S.C., J.G., A.L., F.D., C.P., G.F. and J.-C.P.; visualization, C.G.; supervision, J.-C.P.; project administration, S.C.; funding acquisition, F.L., I.T., B.C., P.B., A.G., P.A., S.C., C.P., G.F. and J.-C.P. All authors have read and agreed to the published version of the manuscript.

Funding: This research was funded by French National Health Insurance (Occupational Risk Prevention Department), French Ministry of Labour and Social Relations, French Agency for Food, Environmental and Occupational Health and Safety (ANSES grant 07-CRD-51, EST 2006/1/43, EST 2009/68).

Institutional Review Board Statement: The study was approved by the hospital ethics committee (CPPRB Paris-Cochin n°1946 (2002), CPP Ile De France III n°1946/11/02-02 (2010)).

Informed Consent Statement: All participants received information about the study and gave their written informed consent.

Data Availability Statement: The data presented in this study are available on request from the corresponding author. The data are not publicly available due to privacy.

Conflicts of Interest: The authors declare no conflict of interest.

References

1. Paris, C.; Thierry, S.; Brochard, P.; Letourneux, M.; Schorlé, E.; Stoufflet, A.; Ameille, J.; Conso, F.; Pairon, J.C.; Members, T.N.A. Pleural plaques and asbestosis: Dose- and time-response relationships based on HRCT data. *Eur. Respir. J.* **2009**, *34*, 72–79. [CrossRef] [PubMed]
2. Aberle, D.R.; Gamsu, G.; Ray, C. High-resolution CT of benign asbestos-related diseases: Clinical and radiographic correlation. *Am. J. Roentgenol.* **1988**, *151*, 883–891. [CrossRef] [PubMed]
3. Gamsu, G.; Aberle, D.R. CT findings in pulmonary asbestosis. *Am. J. Roentgenol.* **1995**, *165*, 486–487. [CrossRef]
4. Staples, C.A.; Gamsu, G.; Ray, C.S.; Webb, W.R. High Resolution Computed Tomography and Lung Function in Asbestos-exposed Workers with Normal Chest Radiographs. *Am. Rev. Respir. Dis.* **1989**, *139*, 1502–1508. [CrossRef]
5. Algranti, E.; Mendonça, E.; DeCapitani, E.; Freitas, J.; Silva, H.; Bussacos, M. Non-malignant asbestos-related diseases in Brazilian asbestos-cement workers. *Am. J. Ind. Med.* **2001**, *40*, 240–254. [CrossRef] [PubMed]
6. Paris, C.; Benichou, J.; Raffaelli, C.; Genevois, A.; Fournier, L.; Menard, G.; Broessel, N.; Ameille, J.; Brochard, P.; Gillon, J.-C.; et al. Factors associated with early-stage pulmonary fibrosis as determined by high-resolution computed tomography among persons occupationally exposed to asbestos. *Scand. J. Work. Environ. Health* **2004**, *30*, 206–214. [CrossRef] [PubMed]
7. Vierikko, T.; Järvenpää, R.; Toivio, P.; Uitti, J.; Oksa, P.; Lindholm, T.; Vehmas, T. Clinical and HRCT screening of heavily asbestos-exposed workers. *Int. Arch. Occup. Environ. Health* **2010**, *83*, 47–54. [CrossRef]
8. Lederer, D.J.; Enright, P.L.; Kawut, S.M.; Hoffman, E.A.; Hunninghake, G.; Van Beek, E.J.R.; Austin, J.H.M.; Jiang, R.; Lovasi, G.S.; Barr, R.G. Cigarette smoking is associated with subclinical parenchymal lung disease: The Multi-Ethnic Study of Atherosclerosis (MESA)-lung study. *Am. J. Respir. Crit. Care Med.* **2009**, *180*, 407–414. [CrossRef]
9. Araki, T.; Putman, R.K.; Hatabu, H.; Gao, W.; Dupuis, J.; Latourelle, J.C.; Nishino, M.; Zazueta, O.E.; Kurugol, S.; Ross, J.C.; et al. Development and Progression of Interstitial Lung Abnormalities in the Framingham Heart Study. *Am. J. Respir. Crit. Care Med.* **2016**, *194*, 1514–1522. [CrossRef] [PubMed]
10. Putman, R.K.; Hatabu, H.; Araki, T.; Gudmundsson, G.; Gao, W.; Nishino, M.; Okajima, Y.; Dupuis, J.; Latourelle, J.C.; Cho, M.H.; et al. Association Between Interstitial Lung Abnormalities and All-Cause Mortality. *JAMA* **2016**, *315*, 672–681. [CrossRef]

11. Copley, S.J.; Wells, A.U.; Hawtin, K.E.; Gibson, D.J.; Hodson, J.M.; Jacques, A.E.T.; Hansell, D.M. Lung Morphology in the Elderly: Comparative CT Study of Subjects over 75 Years Old versus Those under 55 Years Old. *Radiology* **2009**, *251*, 566–573. [CrossRef]
12. Washko, G.R.; Hunninghake, G.M.; Fernandez, I.E.; Nishino, M.; Okajima, Y.; Yamashiro, T.; Ross, J.C.; Estépar, R.S.J.; Lynch, D.A.; Brehm, J.; et al. Lung Volumes and Emphysema in Smokers with Interstitial Lung Abnormalities. *New Engl. J. Med.* **2011**, *364*, 897–906. [CrossRef]
13. Sverzellati, N.; Guerci, L.; Randi, G.; Calabro, E.; La Vecchia, C.; Marchianò, A.; Pesci, A.; Zompatori, M.; Pastorino, U. Interstitial lung diseases in a lung cancer screening trial. *Eur. Respir. J.* **2011**, *38*, 392–400. [CrossRef]
14. Hunninghake, G.M.; Hatabu, H.; Okajima, Y.; Gao, W.; Dupuis, J.; Latourelle, J.; Nishino, M.; Araki, T.; Zazueta, O.E.; Kurugol, S.; et al. MUC5B Promoter Polymorphism and Interstitial Lung Abnormalities. *New Engl. J. Med.* **2013**, *368*, 2192–2200. [CrossRef]
15. Putman, R.K.; Gudmundsson, G.; Axelsson, G.T.; Hida, T.; Honda, O.; Araki, T.; Yanagawa, M.; Nishino, M.; Miller, E.R.; Eiriksdottir, G.; et al. Imaging Patterns Are Associated with Interstitial Lung Abnormality Progression and Mortality. *Am. J. Respir. Crit. Care Med.* **2019**, *200*, 175–183. [CrossRef] [PubMed]
16. Ameille, J.; Letourneux, M.; Paris, C.; Brochard, P.; Stoufflet, A.; Schorlé, E.; Gislard, A.; Laurent, F.; Conso, F.; Pairon, J.-C. Does Asbestos Exposure Cause Airway Obstruction, in the Absence of Confirmed Asbestosis? *Am. J. Respir. Crit. Care Med.* **2010**, *182*, 526–530. [CrossRef] [PubMed]
17. Clin, B.; Luc, A.; Morlais, F.; Paris, C.; Ameille, J.; Brochard, P.; De Girolamo, J.; Gislard, A.; Laurent, F.; Letourneux, M.; et al. Pulmonary nodules detected by thoracic computed tomography scan after exposure to asbestos: Diagnostic significance. *Int. J. Tuberc. Lung Dis.* **2011**, *15*, 1707–1714. [CrossRef]
18. Pairon, J.-C.; Laurent, F.; Rinaldo, M.; Clin, B.; Andujar, P.; Ameille, J.; Brochard, P.; Chammings, S.; Ferretti, G.; Salle, F.G.; et al. Pleural Plaques and the Risk of Pleural Mesothelioma. *J. Natl. Cancer Inst.* **2013**, *105*, 293–301. [CrossRef] [PubMed]
19. Hansell, D.M.; Bankier, A.A.; MacMahon, H.; McLoud, T.C.; Müller, N.L.; Remy, J. Fleischner Society: Glossary of Terms for Thoracic Imaging. *Radiology* **2008**, *246*, 697–722. [CrossRef]
20. Raghu, G.; Collard, H.R.; Egan, J.J.; Martinez, F.J.; Behr, J.; Brown, K.K.; Colby, T.V.; Cordier, J.-F.; Flaherty, K.R.; Lasky, J.A.; et al. An Official ATS/ERS/JRS/ALAT Statement: Idiopathic Pulmonary Fibrosis: Evidence-based Guidelines for Diagnosis and Management. *Am. J. Respir. Crit. Care Med.* **2011**, *183*, 788–824. [CrossRef]
21. Royston, P. A strategy for modelling the effect of a continuous covariate in medicine and epidemiology. *Stat. Med.* **2000**, *19*, 1831–1847. [CrossRef]
22. Vehmas, T.; Kivisaari, L.; Huuskonen, M.S.; Jaakkola, M.S. Scoring CT/HRCT findings among asbestos-exposed workers: Effects of patient's age, body mass index and common laboratory test results. *Eur. Radiol.* **2004**, *15*, 213–219. [CrossRef] [PubMed]
23. Raghu, G.; Remy-Jardin, M.; Myers, J.L.; Richeldi, L.; Ryerson, C.J.; Lederer, D.J.; Behr, J.; Cottin, V.; Danoff, S.K.; Morell, F.; et al. Diagnosis of Idiopathic Pulmonary Fibrosis. An Official ATS/ERS/JRS/ALAT Clinical Practice Guideline. *Am. J. Respir. Crit. Care Med.* **2018**, *198*, e44–e68. [CrossRef] [PubMed]
24. Hansell, D.M. Thin-Section CT of the Lungs: The Hinterland of Normal. *Radiology* **2010**, *256*, 695–711. [CrossRef]
25. Jin, G.Y.; Lynch, D.; Chawla, A.; Garg, K.; Tammemagi, M.C.; Sahin, H.; Misumi, S.; Kwon, K.S. Interstitial lung abnormalities in a CT lung cancer screening population: Prevalence and progression rate. *Radiology* **2013**, *268*, 563–571. [CrossRef]
26. Copley, S.J.; Wells, A.U.; Sivakumaran, P.; Rubens, M.B.; Lee, Y.C.G.; Desai, S.; Macdonald, S.L.S.; Thompson, R.I.; Colby, T.V.; Nicholson, A.G.; et al. Asbestosis and Idiopathic Pulmonary Fibrosis: Comparison of Thin-Section CT Features. *Radiology* **2003**, *229*, 731–736. [CrossRef] [PubMed]
27. Laurent, F.; Paris, C.; Ferretti, G.; Beigelman-Aubry, C.; Montaudon, M.; Latrabe, V.; Jankowski, A.; Badachi, Y.; Clin, B.; Gislard, A.; et al. Inter-reader agreement in HRCT detection of pleural plaques and asbestosis in participants with previous occupational exposure to asbestos. *Occup. Environ. Med.* **2014**, *71*, 865–870. [CrossRef] [PubMed]
28. Baumgartner, K.B.; Samet, J.M.; Stidley, C.A.; Colby, T.V.; Waldron, J.A. Cigarette smoking: A risk factor for idiopathic pulmonary fibrosis. *Am. J. Respir. Crit. Care Med.* **1997**, *155*, 242–248. [CrossRef]
29. Huuskonen, O.; Kivisaari, L.; Zitting, A.; Kaleva, S.; Vehmas, T. Emphysema findings associated with heavy asbestos-exposure in high resolution computed tomography of finnish construction workers. *J. Occup. Health* **2004**, *46*, 266–271. [CrossRef] [PubMed]

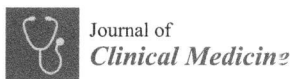

Article

Compressed Sensing Real-Time Cine Reduces CMR Arrhythmia-Related Artifacts

Benjamin Longère [1,*], Paul-Edouard Allard [2], Christos V Gkizas [2], Augustin Coisne [1], Justin Hennicaux [2], Arianna Simeone [2], Michaela Schmidt [3], Christoph Forman [3], Solenn Toupin [4], David Montaigne [1] and François Pontana [1]

1. University of Lille, Inserm, CHU Lille, Institut Pasteur Lille, U1011—European Genomic Institute for Diabetes (EGID), F-59000 Lille, France; augustin.coisne@chru-lille.fr (A.C.); david.montaigne@chru-lille.fr (D.M.); francois.pontana@chru-lille.fr (F.P.)
2. CHU Lille, Department of Cardiovascular Radiology, F-59000 Lille, France; pauledouard.allard@chru-lille.fr (P.-E.A.); chgkizas@gmail.com (C.V.G.); justin.hennicaux@chru-lille.fr (J.H.); arianna.simeone@chru-lille.fr (A.S.)
3. MR Product Innovation and Definition, Magnetic Resonance, Siemens Healthcare GmbH, 91052 Erlangen, Germany; michaela.schmidt@siemens-healthineers.com (M.S.); christoph.forman@siemens-healthineers.com (C.F.)
4. Scientific Partnerships, Siemens Healthcare France, 93200 Saint-Denis, France; solenn.toupin@siemens-healthineers.com
* Correspondence: benjamin.longere@chru-lille.fr

Citation: Longère, B.; Allard, P.-E.; Gkizas, C.V.; Coisne, A.; Hennicaux, J.; Simeone, A.; Schmidt, M.; Forman, C.; Toupin, S.; Montaigne, D.; et al. Compressed Sensing Real-Time Cine Reduces CMR Arrhythmia-Related Artifacts. *J. Clin. Med.* **2021**, *10*, 3274. https://doi.org/10.3390/jcm10153274

Academic Editor: Mickaël Ohana

Received: 22 June 2021
Accepted: 21 July 2021
Published: 24 July 2021

Publisher's Note: MDPI stays neutral with regard to jurisdictional claims in published maps and institutional affiliations.

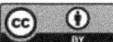

Copyright: © 2021 by the authors. Licensee MDPI, Basel, Switzerland. This article is an open access article distributed under the terms and conditions of the Creative Commons Attribution (CC BY) license (https://creativecommons.org/licenses/by/4.0/).

Abstract: Background and objective: Cardiac magnetic resonance (CMR) is a key tool for cardiac work-up. However, arrhythmia can be responsible for arrhythmia-related artifacts (ARA) and increased scan time using segmented sequences. The aim of this study is to evaluate the effect of cardiac arrhythmia on image quality in a comparison of a compressed sensing real-time (CS_{rt}) cine sequence with the reference prospectively gated segmented balanced steady-state free precession ($Cine_{ref}$) technique regarding ARA. Methods: A total of 71 consecutive adult patients (41 males; mean age = 59.5 ± 20.1 years (95% CI: 54.7–64.2 years)) referred for CMR examination with concomitant irregular heart rate (defined by an RR interval coefficient of variation >10%) during scanning were prospectively enrolled. For each patient, two cine sequences were systematically acquired: first, the reference prospectively triggered multi-breath-hold $Cine_{ref}$ sequence including a short-axis stack, one four-chamber slice, and a couple of two-chamber slices; second, an additional single breath-hold CS_{rt} sequence providing the same slices as the reference technique. Two radiologists independently assessed ARA and image quality (overall, acquisition, and edge sharpness) for both techniques. Results: The mean heart rate was 71.8 ± 19.0 (SD) beat per minute (bpm) (95% CI: 67.4–76.3 bpm) and its coefficient of variation was 25.0 ± 9.4 (SD) % (95% CI: 22.8–27.2%). Acquisition was significantly faster with CS_{rt} than with $Cine_{ref}$ ($Cine_{ref}$: 556.7 ± 143.4 (SD) s (95% CI: 496.7–616.7 s); CS_{rt}: 23.9 ± 7.9 (SD) s (95% CI: 20.6–27.1 s); $p < 0.0001$). A total of 595 pairs of cine slices were evaluated (median: 8 (range: 6–14) slices per patient). The mean proportion of ARA-impaired slices per patient was 85.9 ± 22.7 (SD) % using $Cine_{ref}$, but this was figure was zero using CS_{rt} ($p < 0.0001$). The European CMR registry artifact score was lower with CS_{rt} (median: 1 (range: 0–5)) than with $Cine_{ref}$ (median: 3 (range: 0–3); $p < 0.0001$). Subjective image quality was higher in CS_{rt} than in $Cine_{ref}$ (median: 3 (range: 1–3) versus 2 (range: 1–4), respectively; $p < 0.0001$). In line, edge sharpness was higher on CS_{rt} cine than on $Cine_{ref}$ images (0.054 ± 0.016 pixel^{-1} (95% CI: 0.050–0.057 pixel^{-1}) versus 0.042 ± 0.022 pixel^{-1} (95% CI: 0.037–0.047 pixel^{-1}), respectively; $p = 0.0001$. Conclusion: Compressed sensing real-time cine drastically reduces arrhythmia-related artifacts and thus improves cine image quality in patients with arrhythmia.

Keywords: cardiac; heart; magnetic resonance; CMR; compressed sensing; real-time; fast imaging; arrhythmia; artifact

1. Introduction

Cardiac magnetic resonance (CMR) is a major imaging modality for the assessment of left and right ventricular volumes and mass [1–3]. Moreover, it provides effective morphologic and kinetic assessment, including of the right ventricle which is not easily evaluated with ultrasounds due to its retrosternal location [4]. Multi-breath-hold segmented balanced steady state free precession (bSSFP) sequences are considered superior to gradient-echo imaging since they provide better endocardium delineation and reproducibility in a shorter scan time [5]. Retrospective electrocardiogram (ECG) gating requires the heart rate (HR) to be a regular periodic phenomenon as pieces of data are continuously acquired on multiple cardiac cycles, time-labelled and merged for the reconstruction of a whole cine slice, which is a weighted representation of successive heartbeats. It allows adapting the length of the acquisition window to the duration of the heartbeat during the continuous acquisition. This enables capturing of the complete cardiac cycle in segmented acquisitions. Typically, k-space interpolation or filtering is applied to retrospectively gate the acquired data to a reference heartbeat [6,7]. In the case of arrhythmia, artifacts occur since reconstruction is performed using incoming data from different frames of the cardiac cycle. Arrhythmia rejection algorithms can be applied with retrospective gating but may end in exceedingly long breath-holds. These arrhythmia-related artifacts (ARA) may be limited using prospectively triggered sequences by setting the acquisition window shorter than the briefest measured RR interval (time laps between two consecutive R peaks) [8]. However, this requires decreasing the number of k-space lines acquired per cardiac frame in order to preserve the widely accepted temporal resolution of 20 phases per cardiac cycle and misses to display the diastolic phases [9,10]. As a result of these adjustments, longer breath-holds and scan time are observed while the last phases of the cardiac cycle are not sampled.

Decreasing the amount of measured data is a simple way to reduce acquisition time. In recent years, compressed sensing was established as a powerful method to drastically reduce scan time [11–14]. This is achieved by highly undersampling k-space with a random sampling pattern. After Fourier transform, these acquired data result in noise-like, incoherent artifacts. These artifacts are compensated for in the final image with a non-linear iterative reconstruction exploiting the fact that medical images have a sparse representation. In combination with parallel imaging, acceleration rates can be achieved with CS that enable real-time cardiac cine imaging based on a balanced bSSFP readout with spatiotemporal resolution in a similar range to the reference ($Cine_{ref}$) acquisitions [15].

Various CMR studies have evaluated real-time CS cine sequences in 1.5 and 3 Tesla magnetic resonance scanners showing promising results for the assessment of left and right ventricles, including in patients with atrial fibrillation [16–21]. However, image quality was not specifically assessed in patients with irregular HR. Based on the assumption that real-time CS cine (CS_{rt}) could reduce ARA, our study aimed at evaluating its image quality as compared to the reference multi-breath-hold segmented bSSFP cine ($Cine_{ref}$) in patients suffering from cardiac arrhythmia.

2. Materials and Methods

2.1. Study Population

From January 2019 to December 2019, 71 adult patients referred to our cardiovascular radiology department for CMR with concomitant arrhythmia during scanning were enrolled. Irregular HR was defined when the coefficient of variation of RR intervals (CV_{RR}) was greater than 10% while scanning. The CV_{RR} was calculated as the ratio of the standard deviation to the mean of RR intervals' durations which were obtained from digital imaging and communications in medicine (DICOM) fields. Patients under 18 years old, grown-up congenital heart disease, stress CMR, patients undergoing ECG retrogated CMR and patients with sinus rhythm were excluded. A graphic illustration of the study design is provided in Figure S1 (Supplementary Materials). The protocol was approved by our institutional ethics committee and patients gave informed consent. The study was approved by the French National Agency for the Safety of Medicines and Health Devices (ANSM; ID-RCB: 2017-A00852-51).

2.2. Imaging Protocol

CMR studies were performed on a 1.5 T scanner (MAGNETOM Aera, Siemens Healthcare, Erlangen, Germany). Every patient underwent two series of cine images: first, the reference prospectively triggered and segmented multi-breath-hold $Cine_{ref}$ sequence; second, the prototype single-breath-hold real-time single-shot CS_{rt} cine sequence. Both acquisitions included one left ventricular (LV) and one right ventricular (RV) two-chamber slice, one four-chamber slice and a LV short-axis stack covering both ventricles with an 8 mm slice thickness and a 2 mm gap. Regarding the prospectively gated $Cine_{ref}$ sequence, 20 phases of the cardiac cycle were acquired and the number of views per frame was set to reach this sampling rate. In single-shot CS_{rt} cine imaging, the data acquisition was performed in a single heartbeat. The acquisition was triggered by the R peak on the ECG. With adaptive triggering, the acquisition was stopped with the next R peak, which allowed capturing the complete cardiac cycle. However, for multi-slice acquisition it could lead to a variation in the number of cardiac phases acquired between different slices as the temporal resolution was fixed. Temporal interpolation was applied to generate an additional dataset with a fixed number of cardiac phases ($n = 20$). This dataset was used to quantify cardiac function using a dedicated post-processing software that required a fixed number of cardiac phases. To evaluate the CS_{rt} sequence in clinical conditions, 40 iterations were used to perform image recovery to maintain an acceptable reconstruction time. An additional phase contrast imaging (PCI) flow sequence was acquired on the aortic root. Segmented $Cine_{ref}$ and CS_{rt} cine sequences parameters are available in Table 1.

Table 1. Imaging parameters of the reference prospectively triggered steady-state free-precession cine imaging and real-time compressed sensing cine imaging.

Parameters	$Cine_{ref}$	CS_{rt}
Repetition time—ms	3.16	2.70
Echo time—ms	1.23	1.14
Flip angle—degrees	57	60
Field of view—mm^2	375 × 280	360 × 270
Matrix—pixels^2	288 × 216	224 × 168
Spatial resolution—mm^2	1.3 × 1.3	1.6 × 1.6
Temporal resolution—ms	41.2	49
Slice thickness/gap—mm	8/2	8/2
Bandwidth—Hz/pixel	915	900
ECG mode	Prospective triggering	Adaptative triggering
Number of measured cardiac phases per cycle	20 [a]	17.0 ± 3.2
Number of reconstructed cardiac frames per cycle—n	20 [a]	20 [b]
Number of views per frame—n	13.0 ± 4.8 [c]	18 [a]
Cycles of iterative reconstruction—n	NA	40
Acceleration factor	2	11

Data are expressed as mean ± standard deviation in the absence of any indication. [a] Constant value. [b] Interpolation was performed to provide a constant frame rate of 20 cardiac phases per cycle for post-processing. [c] The number of views per frame was set according to the shorter RR interval in order to acquire 20 cardiac phases. Prospective triggering allows data sampling during a fixed acquisition window after each R peak while adaptative triggering allow data sampling until the next R peak occurs. Abbreviations: $Cine_{ref}$, reference segmented cine; CS_{rt}, real-time compressed sensing cine; ECG, electrocardiogram; n, data represented as numbers; NA, not applicable.

2.3. Cine Images Quality Assessment

Image quality was evaluated in both groups using four indicators. First, the subjective overall image quality was evaluated using a subjective 4-point Likert scale (1: non diagnostic; 2: poor; 3: good; 4: excellent). Secondly, an objective image quality assessment was carried out based on standardized criteria adapted from the European CMR registry

"LV-Function cine SSFP" section (referred to below as "EuroCMR score") [22] (p. 3). Higher scores referred to more frequent artifact occurrence (Table 2).

Table 2. "LV-Function cine SSFP" section of the standardized objective quality criteria score based on the European CMR registry. Adapted from [22] (p. 3).

Items	0	1	2	3	Maximum Score
1. LV coverage	Full	-	No apex	Base or ≥1 slice missing	5
2. Wrap around	No	1 slice	2 slices	≥3 slices	
3. Respiratory ghost	No	1 slice	2 slices	≥3 slices	
4. Cardiac ghost	No	1 slice	2 slices	≥3 slices	3
5. Blurring/ARA	No	1 slice	2 slices	≥3 slices	
6. Metallic artifacts	No	1 slice	2 slices	≥3 slices	
7. Shimming artifacts	No	1 slice	2 slices	≥3 slices	
8. Signal loss (coil inactive)	Activated	-	Not activated		2
9. Orientation of stack	Correct	-	Incorrect	-	2
10. Slice thickness	≤10 mm	11–15 mm	-	>15 mm	3
11. Gap	≤3 mm	3–4 mm	-	>4 mm	3
12. Correct LV long axes	≥2 mm	1	-	None	3
Score					21
Modified score (items 1 to 8)					**10**

Every acquisition using both sequences marked a null score concerning the four last items. Indeed, acquisitions were repeated every time slice orientation was not appropriated (item 9 = 0); all acquisitions (Cine$_{ref}$ and CS$_{rt}$) were performed using the same slice thickness and gap which were 8 mm (item 10 = 0) and 2 mm (item 11 = 0), respectively, and both horizontal and vertical long-axis slices were systematically acquired (item 12 = 0). Criteria in italics were not applied, and only bold criteria were used for objective quality assessment in our study, providing a maximum score of 10 points. The more artifacts there were, the higher the score was. Abbreviations: LV, left ventricle; SSFP, steady-state free precession; CMR, cardiac magnetic resonance; Cine$_{ref}$, reference segmented cine; CS$_{rt}$, real-time compressed sensing cine; ARA, arrhythmia-related artifacts.

Third, the proportion of short-axis slices affected by ARA in each stack of both sequences was calculated, referred to as ARA rate. ARA were defined as a blurring of all or a part of the LV wall borders [22].

Finally, the edge sharpness (ε) of the boundary between myocardium and blood pool, which is the spatial frequency (in pixel^{-1}) reflecting the spatial resolution, was measured on paired Cine$_{ref}$ and CS$_{rt}$ four-chamber slices at end-diastole, accordingly to the literature [23,24]. Additional measurement at end-systole was performed. The edge spread function (ESF), which is the response of the imaging system to a high contrast boundary, was measured on MATLAB (version R2015a, The MathWorks, Natick, MA, USA), by drawing a signal profile line perpendicularly across the edge between the interventricular septum and the LV blood pool (Figure 1a,b) [25]. Then, ε was calculated as the reciprocal of the distance separating the points corresponding to 20% and 80% of the difference between local minimum and maximum signal intensities (Figure 1c,d).

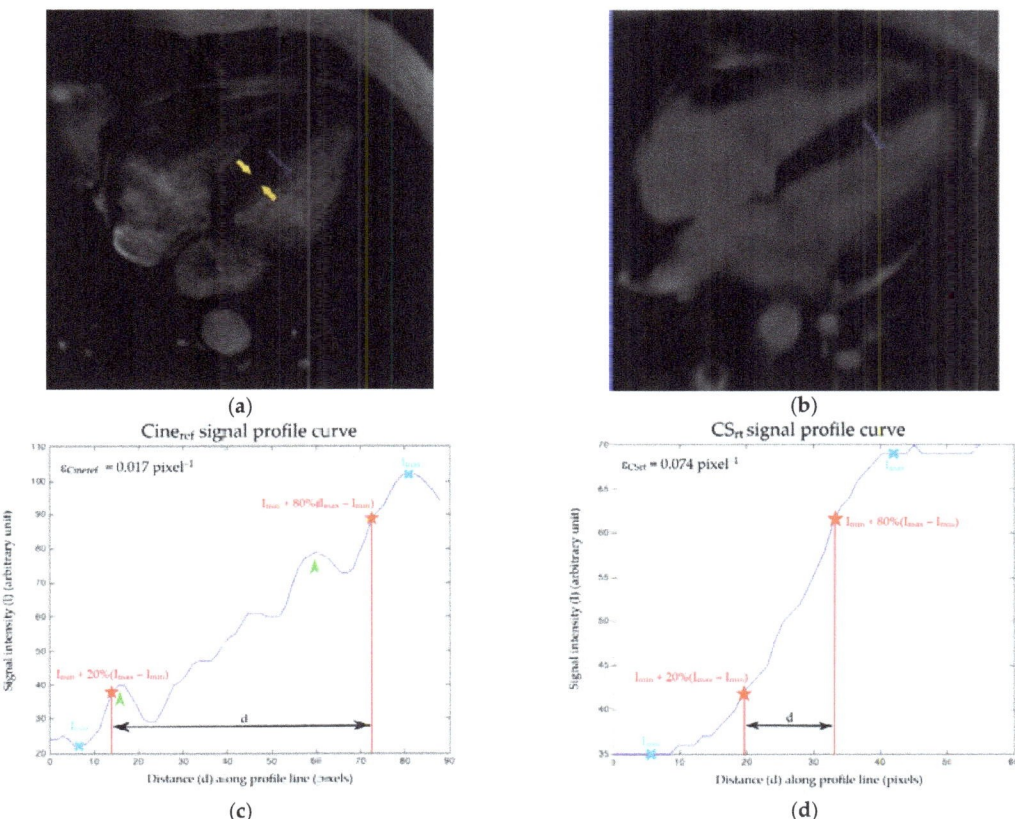

Figure 1. Example of edge sharpness assessment at end-diastole for a 56-year-old male patient suffering from atrial fibrillation. The same four-chamber view at end-diastole is acquired with (**a**) the $Cine_{ref}$ sequence and (**b**) the CS_{rt} sequence. An orthogonal profile line was drawn at mid-cavity across the border between the septal myocardium and the left ventricular blood pool (blue line) on a four-chamber view. It provided intensity profiles (blue curves) along the line for (**c**) $Cine_{ref}$ and (**d**) CS_{rt} cine. The edge sharpness was the inverse of the distance d (in pixels) between the positions corresponding to 20% and 80% (red stars) of the difference between the maximum and minimum signal intensities (blue crosses). The edge sharpness was expressed in $pixel^{-1}$. This measurement was performed at end-diastole and end-systole for both sequences. Note that the peaks (arrows heads) added to the $Cine_{ref}$ signal profile curve (**c**) correspond to the doubling of the interventricular septum border (arrows) on the cine view (**a**). The same assessment was performed on both sequences at end-diastole and end-systole for the 71 enrolled patients. Abbreviations: $Cine_{ref}$, reference segmented cine; CS_{rt}, real-time compressed sensing cine; $\varepsilon_{Cineref}$, edge sharpness measured on $Cine_{ref}$ sequence; ε_{CSrt}, edge sharpness measured on CS_{rt} cine; I, signal intensity; I_{min}, minimal signal intensity; I_{max}, maximal signal intensity; d, distance along the profile line.

2.4. Conditions of Image Analysis

Images from both sequences were anonymized before transfer to a clinical workstation (Sygno.via VB30A, Siemens Healthcare, Erlangen, Germany). A radiologist with 4 years of experience (PEA) performed the image quality assessment according to the above-cited indicators. Image sets were randomly evaluated in each group. The same observer (PEA) first performed the quality assessment of the reference $Cine_{ref}$ images and at least one month later evaluated the CS_{rt} images. For each patient, arrhythmia was quantified by calculating the CV_{RR}. An additional assessment was performed by a radiologist with 8 years of experience (BL) from 30 randomly selected patients to evaluate the interobserver agreement and performed the same assessment regarding subjective quality, EuroCMR score and ARA rates. In the case of mismatch between the two readers, a radiologist with 15 years of experience (FP) performed the quality assessment with the two others to reach consensual scores which were used instead of those set by the first and less experienced observer. Mismatches were defined by discrepancies greater than or equal to 2 points regarding subjective quality score and EuroCMR score, or by a 20% difference in ARA rates. The edge sharpness assessment was automated and was not evaluated for interobserver agreement. Finally, semi-automated segmentation of LV endocardium and epicardium, and manual segmentation RV endocardium were performed on the same workstation with both cine sequences for each patient. LV stroke volume was also measured on PCI sequence.

2.5. Statistics Analysis

Categorical data were represented as numbers (percentages), continuous variables as mean ± standard deviation (SD) (95% confidence interval (CI)) in case of normal distribution and median (range: minimum–maximum) in other cases. Sequences were compared using the Wilcoxon signed-rank test regarding the overall subjective quality score and the modified EuroCMR score. Paired Student's t-test was used for ARA rates, edge sharpness comparisons, and ventricular functional parameters comparison. An analysis of variance (ANOVA) was used to compare LV stroke volumes assessed by cine segmentation and PCI flow sequence. Intraclass correlation coefficient and kappa test were applied to assess the interobserver agreement [26]. Values of $p < 0.05$ were considered statistically significant. Statistical analysis was performed using MedCalc software (version 14.8.1.0, MedCalc Software, Ostend, Belgium).

3. Results

3.1. Population Description

The mean age of the population was 59.5 ± 20.1 (SD) years (95% CI: 54.7–64.2 years) with a male predominance ($n = 41/71$; 57.7%, women: $n = 30/71$; 42.3%). Patients were referred for initial work-up or follow-up of coronary artery disease ($n = 17$; 23.9%), heart rhythm disorder ($n = 14$; 19.7%), dilated cardiomyopathy ($n = 11$; 15.5%), infiltrative cardiomyopathy ($n = 8$; 11.3%), heart valve disease ($n = 7$; 9.9%), myocarditis ($n = 6$; 8.5%), hypertrophic cardiomyopathy ($n = 5$; 7.0%), and heart failure ($n = 3$; 4.2%). The mean HR was 71.8 ± 19.0 beats per minute (bpm) (95% CI: 67.4–76.3 bpm) and 38.0% of the patients ($n = 27/71$) demonstrated a mean HR above 75 bpm, meaning the 49 ms temporal resolution of the CS_{rt} cine provided less than 16 frames of the cardiac cycle per slice. The mean CV_{RR} was 25.0 ± 9.4% (95% CI: 22.8–27.2%). Arrhythmia was caused by atrial fibrillation ($n = 42/71$; 59.2%), ventricular hyperexcitability ($n = 17/71$; 23.9%), and conduction disorders ($n = 12/71$; 16.9%). Demographic data are summarized in Table 3. Biventricular functional assessment of the population is reported in Table 4.

Table 3. Study population characteristics.

	Mean ± SD (95% CI)	Minimum Value	Maximum Value
Age—years	59.5 ± 20.1 (54.7–64.2)	18	87
Height—cm	171.6 ± 9.1 (169.4–173.7)	140	188
Weight—kg	79.3 ± 19.5 (74.7–83.9)	26	131
Body mass index—kg/m^2	26.8 ± 6.1 (25.4–28.3)	13.3	47.0
Maximal heart rate—bpm	85.9 ± 21.6 (80.8–91.0)	50	139
Minimal heart rate—bpm	55.6 ± 18.7 (55.6–64.4)	31	107
Mean heart rate—bpm	71.8 ± 19.0 (67.4–76.3)	42	116
Arrhythmia (CV_{RR})—%	25.0 ± 9.4 (22.8–27.2)	10.2	50.9

Abbreviations: CV_{RR}, coefficient of variation of RR interval; bpm, beat per minute; SD, standard deviation; 95% CI, 95% confidence interval.

Table 4. Biventricular functional assessment of the study population.

	Cine$_{ref}$	CS$_{rt}$	Difference	PCI	p
LVEF—%	47.7 ± 19.0 (39.9–55.6)	47.3 ± 18.9 (39.5–55.1)	−0.4 ± 1.9 (−1.2 to 0.4)	-	0.30 [a]
LVEDV—mL	193.2 ± 102.0 (151.1–235.3)	189.6 ± 101.9 (147.6–231.6)	−3.6 ± 7.2 (−6.5 to −0.6)	-	0.02 [a]
LVESV—mL	114.2 ± 99.8 (73.0–155.4)	113.3 ± 98.8 (72.5–154.1)	−0.9 ± 6.8 (−3.7 to 1.9)	-	0.51 [a]
LVSV—mL	79.0 ± 29.4 (66.9–91.1)	76.3 ± 28.7 (64.5–88.2)	-	76.7 ± 30.1 (64.3–89.1)	0.94 [b]
LVM—g	145.2 ± 48.0 (125.4–165.1)	148.0 ± 50.1 (127.3–168.6)	2.7 ± 8.8 (−0.9 to 6.3)	-	0.13 [a]
RVEF—%	50.9 ± 11.9 (46.0–55.8)	51.8 ± 11.9 (46.9–56.7)	0.9 ± 1.8 (0.1 to 1.7)	-	0.02 [a]
RVEDV—mL	153.7 ± 52.1 (132.2–175.2)	148.4 ± 47.5 (128.8–168.0)	−5.3 ± 7.6 (−8.5 to −2.2)	-	0.02 [a]
RVESV—mL	77.5 ± 38.0 (61.8–93.1)	73.8 ± 36.1 (58.9–88.7)	−3.7 ± 5.8 (−6.1 to −1.3)	-	0.004 [a]
RVSV—mL	76.2 ± 27.3 (65.0–87.5)	74.6 ± 24.1 (64.6–84.5)	−1.7 ± 4.5 (−3.5 to 0.2)	Insufficient data	0.08 [a]

Data are presented as mean ± SD (95% CI). The significance of statistic tests is defined by values of $p < 0.05$. [a] Student's t-test; [b] Analysis of variance. Abbreviations: Cine$_{ref}$, reference segmented cine; CS$_{rt}$, real-time compressed sensing cine; PCI, phase contrast imaging sequence; SD, standard deviation; 95% CI, 95% confidence interval; LV, left ventricular; RV, right ventricular; EF, ejection fraction; EDV, end-diastolic volume; ESV, end-systolic volume; SV, stroke volume; LVM, left ventricular mass

3.2. Cine Acquisitions

A total of 599 short-axis cine slices were acquired with each sequence. A median number of 8 (range: 6–14) cine slices was acquired twice for each patient, depending on cardiac morphology. To acquire the same slices, CS$_{rt}$ was significantly faster than Cine$_{ref}$ (Cine$_{ref}$: 556.7 ± 145.4 (SD) s (95% CI: 496.7–616.7 s); CS$_{rt}$: 23.9 ± 7.9 (SD) s (95% CI: 20.6–27.1 s); $p < 0.0001$).

3.3. Objective European CMR Standardized Criteria-Based Quality Score

The EuroCMR score for the CS$_{rt}$ cine (median: 1 (range: 0–5)) was significantly better than for the Cine$_{ref}$ sequence (median: 3 (range: 0–3); $p < 0.0001$) (Table 5) (Figure 2; Video S1 (Supplementary Materials)). Interobserver agreements were 0.94 and 0.89 regarding Cine$_{ref}$ and CS$_{rt}$, respectively. No mismatch was encountered between the readers.

Table 5. Objective image quality with EuroCMR criteria scores: comparison between Cine$_{ref}$ and CS$_{rt}$ image sets.

Objective European CMR Criteria Scores		CS$_{rt}$					Median (Range)
		0	1–3	4–6	7–10	Total	
Cine$_{ref}$	0	1	1	0	0	2	
	1–3	25	42	2	0	69	
	4–6	0	0	0	0	0	1 (0–5)
	7–10	0	0	0	0	0	
	Total	26	43	2	0	71	
Median (range)			3 (0–3)				$p < 0.0001$

The significance of Wilcoxon signed-rank test is defined by values of $p < 0.05$. Red values represent patients for whom CS$_{rt}$ score was equivalent to or better than that of Cine$_{ref}$ for $n = 68/71$ patients (95.8%). Abbreviations: CMR, cardiac magnetic resonance; Cine$_{ref}$, reference segmented cine; CS$_{rt}$, real-time compressed sensing cine; EuroCMR, European CMR registry.

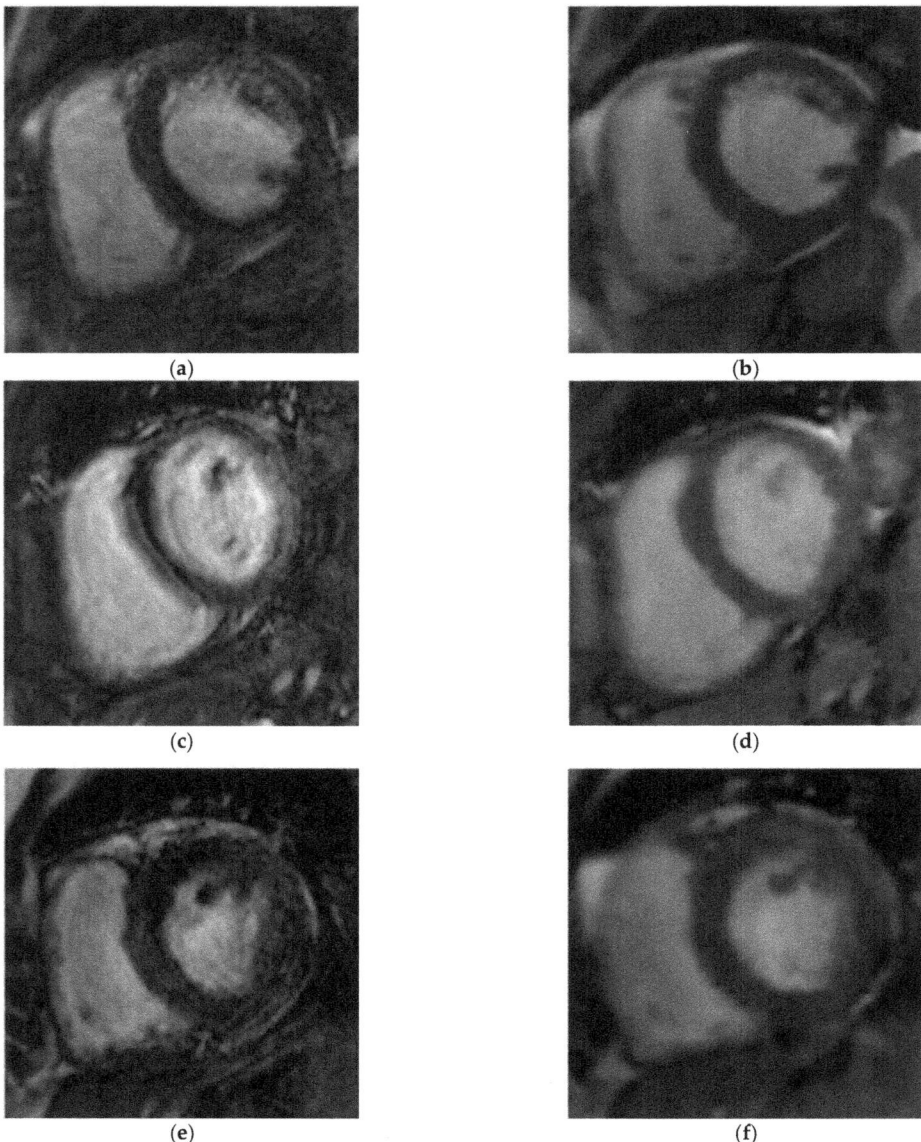

Figure 2. Examples of comparisons between Cine$_{ref}$ and CS$_{rt}$ sequences in three patients suffering from arrhythmia. Mid-cavity short-axis views acquired with (**a,c,e**) Cine$_{ref}$ and (**b,d,f**) CS$_{rt}$. The three patients were (**a,b**) a 74-year-old man suffering from atrial fibrillation, (**c,d**) a 37-year-old woman screened for a genetically proven arrhythmogenic right ventricular cardiomyopathy, (**e,f**) a 63-year-old woman scanned for a second-degree atrioventricular block. The image quality assessment demonstrated: (**a**) Likert scale = 1/4, EuroCMR score = 3/10, $\varepsilon_{Cineref}$ = 0.051 pixel^{-1}; (**b**) Likert scale = 3/4, EuroCMR score = 0/10, ε_{CSrt} = 0.067 pixel^{-1}; (**c**) Likert scale = 1/4, EuroCMR score = 3/10, $\varepsilon_{Cineref}$ = 0.015 pixel^{-1}; (**d**) Likert scale = 3/4, EuroCMR score = 1/10, ε_{CSrt} = 0.050 pixel^{-1}; (**e**) Likert scale = 1/4, EuroCMR score = 3/10, $\varepsilon_{Cineref}$ = 0.023 pixel^{-1}; (**f**) Likert scale = 3/4, EuroCMR score = 0/10, ε_{CSrt} = 0.035 pixel^{-1}. Abbreviations: Cine$_{ref}$, reference segmented cine; CS$_{rt}$, real-time compressed sensing cine; $\varepsilon_{Cineref}$, edge sharpness measured on Cine$_{ref}$; ε_{CSrt}, edge sharpness measured on CS$_{rt}$ cine; EuroCMR, European cardiac magnetic resonance registry.

3.4. Subjective Overall Quality Score

The subjective quality score was significantly better ($p < 0.0001$) for the CS_{rt} sequence with a median score of 3 (range: 1–3). A 0.85 interobserver agreement was reached. The $Cine_{ref}$ sequence provided a median score of 2 (range: 1–4; $p < 0.0001$) with an intraclass coefficient of 0.82 (Table 6). No mismatch was encountered between the readers. The $Cine_{ref}$ sequence provided 23 non-diagnostic acquisitions compromising functional and morphological assessments versus only 10 stacks with the CS_{rt} cine (Figure 2; Video S1 (Supplementary Materials)).

Table 6. Subjective overall image quality scores: comparison between $Cine_{ref}$ and CS_{rt} image sets.

Subjective Overall Quality Scores		CS_{rt}					Median (Range)
		1	2	3	4	Total	
$Cine_{ref}$	1	5	3	15	0	23	
	2	5	6	21	0	32	
	3	0	2	13	0	15	3 (1–3)
	4	0	0	1	0	1	
	Total	10	11	50	0	71	
Median (range)			2 (1–4)				$p < 0.0001$

The significance of Wilcoxon signed-rank test is defined by values of $p < 0.05$. Red values represent patients for whom CS_{rt} score was equivalent to or better than that of $Cine_{ref}$ for $n = 64/71$ patients (90.1%). Abbreviations: $Cine_{ref}$, reference segmented cine; CS_{rt}, real-time compressed sensing cine.

3.5. Arrhythmia-Related Artifacts Rate

ARA using $Cine_{ref}$ sequence were assessed on $n = 514/599$ (85.8%) cine slices from $n = 70/71$ (98.6%) patients, with a 0.90 interobserver agreement. One mismatch was encountered between the readers (PEA: $n = 8/14$, 57.1%; BL: $n = 12/14$, 85.7%; FP: $n = 12/14$, 85.7%). The mean proportion of impaired slices per patient was in 85.9 ± 22.7 (SD) %. No ARA could be depicted using the CS_{rt} sequence.

3.6. Edge Sharpness

The CS_{rt} sequence provided a higher edge sharpness coefficient at end-diastole ($\varepsilon_{CSrt} = 0.051 \pm 0.016$ pixel^{-1} (95% CI: 0.048–0.055 pixel^{-1})) than the $Cine_{ref}$ ($\varepsilon_{Cineref} = 0.040 \pm 0.018$ pixel^{-1} (95% CI: 0.036–0.044 pixel^{-1})) ($p = 0.0001$). A similar finding was observed at end-systole ($\varepsilon_{CSrt} = 0.054 \pm 0.016$ pixel^{-1} (95% CI: 0.050–0.057 pixel^{-1}); $\varepsilon_{Cineref} = 0.042 \pm 0.022$ pixel^{-1} (95% CI: 0.037–0.047 pixel^{-1}); $p = 0.0001$).

4. Discussion

This prospective monocentric study based on a 71-patient cohort is, to our knowledge, the widest and most comprehensive study to evaluate the CS_{rt} sequence in patients with irregular HR. Previous studies in non-selected patients confirmed that real-time CS cine imaging is a reliable alternative to segmented multi-breath-hold SSFP for the assessment of both ventricles' volumes and function in addition to reducing acquisition time [15–20]. Our study demonstrates a dramatic drop in ARA and a significant improvement of subjective and objective image quality with CS_{rt} in patients suffering from heart rhythm disorders. However, no CS_{rt} set was rated as excellent because of the smooth boundaries rendered by the interpolation process which are mandatory for post-processing. Indeed, since the temporal resolution of the CS sequence is fixed, a variable number of frames will be acquired from one cycle to another in the case of arrhythmia. For segmentation to be achieved, post-processing tools require all cine slices to display the same number of frames per cycle. Consequently, a standardization is performed to display 20 frames per cycle on all slices.

We previously showed on a small sub-group of 25 patients suffering from arrhythmia that CS_{rt} and $Cine_{ref}$ sequences allowed similar image quality [20]. However, the present study does not only suggest equivalent scores but significantly better objective and subjective image quality scores with the CS_{rt} cine. Of note, this sequence still provided non-null EuroCMR scores since the slices were identically located on both sequences; accordingly, most of the wrap-around or metallic artifacts were reproduced on the CS_{rt} acquisition.

Our results are in line with the previous study by Goebel et al. on 20 patients with atrial fibrillation [21]. This study focused on a subjective semi-quantitative 4-point quality score and the evaluation of the variation of the myocardial signal intensity which is the reciprocal of the signal-to-noise ratio (SNR). However, this last parameter, or its reciprocal, is considered as hardly suitable for non-linear iterative reconstructions. Moreover, CS is built to suppress pieces of the image signal, while SNR is suited for fully sampled data [27]. Besides our study being specifically designed to evaluate the image quality using additional quantitative and objective metrics, we also performed a clinically integrated evaluation in a larger population.

The higher edge sharpness of CS_{rt} images reflected the faster signal variation along a distance and a better delineation of the image boundaries. We evaluated the edge sharpness both at end-diastole, when the myocardium is supposed to be relatively still, and at end-systole. This metric, regardless of the non-linearity of the reconstruction process, is more suitable than the SNR or its reciprocal to evaluate image quality [27]. The ESF and its inverse value ε measure the imaging system ability to restitute high contrast transition in images. This parameter, the derivative (the line spread function) and its Fourier transform (the so-called task-based modulation transfer function or task transfer function) are currently considered for image quality assessment in the field of non-linear image reconstructions [24,25,28].

Regarding volumetric evaluation in patients suffering from arrhythmia, CS_{rt} provided significantly lower LV end-diastolic volume (−3.6 ± 7.2 mL) than measured on $Cine_{ref}$, which was already observed in previous studies [16,20]. As for RV, there was a significant underestimation of all evaluated functional parameters. Nevertheless, these variations compared to the conventional $Cine_{ref}$ should be considered with caution in a population with arrhythmia. Indeed, irregular heartbeats induce variable ventricular preloads and contractions, making the real reference values impossible to determine. Moreover, since CS_{rt} demonstrated a better image quality than $Cine_{ref}$ that was impaired by ARA, one may consider the segmentation to be more reliable on CS_{rt}.

Besides the image quality improvement, the single breath-hold CS_{rt} sequence allowed a dramatic reduction in scan time. Not only was acquisition faster, but the ARA reduction avoided repeating the acquisition of non-diagnostic slices [20]. The workflow improvement being a major issue in the field of CMR, this real-time sequence is very promising and may improve cost-effectiveness [29].

Limitations

Although the overall subjective image quality was improved with CS_{rt} cine, 10 stacks were still considered as non-diagnostic. Indeed, iterative reconstructions occasionally failed or were not completely achieved on this prototype sequence. Nevertheless, such failures are now rare since the release of the final version of the sequence. Moreover, ECG-related issues occurred when R peaks were occasionally missed, which made the system consider two consecutive heartbeats as one single cycle. The corresponding slices then display a double heart cycle which could not be used for post-processing and was ranked as non-diagnostic. Special attention should be paid to skin preparation before ECG electrode placement.

Other fast real-time sequences, such as radial acquisition, have previously been reported [30,31]. Our study does not compare CS_{rt} to other types of real-time sequences. To our knowledge, no such evaluation has been published and further study would be required for comparison.

A methodological limitation of our study is the impossibility to perform blinded evaluation of the sequences since CS_{rt} cine displayed smoother boundaries than $Cine_{ref}$ sequence. Consequently, observers could recognize the type of sequence they were evaluating. However, paired CS_{rt} and $Cine_{ref}$ stacks from the same patients were separated, randomized, and assessed during different sessions.

Regarding the sampling of heart cycles for the assessment of ventricular volumes and mass, the fixed temporal resolution leads to variable sampling rates from shorter cycler to longer ones. As a consequence, in the case of HR faster than 60 bpm, the recommended 20 frames per cycle could not be acquired [9,10]. However, in the field of analog-to-digital signal conversion, a 16-time oversampling is reputed sufficient for the signal restitution to be accurate, corresponding to a 75 bpm HR [32]. High CV_{RR} in HR may be encountered, and some slices may display undersampled heart cycles. In our study, 38% of the patients demonstrated a mean HR above 75 bpm for whom the undersampling of the cardiac cycle should be considered cautiously during interpretation, especially for volume segmentations. Nevertheless, it must be balanced by the reduction of ARA provided by CS_{rt}.

5. Conclusions

In addition to reducing acquisition time, CS_{rt} sequence drastically reduces arrhythmia-related artifacts and improves image quality in patients with irregular heart rate. This rapid imaging technique allows practitioners, in daily practice, to improve quality, workflow and accessibility of CMR for patients with challenging cardiac conditions.

Supplementary Materials: The following are available online at https://www.mdpi.com/article/10.3390/jcm10153274/s1, Figure S1: Study design. Video S1: Viability assessment in a 77-year-old man with premature ventricular contractions caused by ischemic scars.

Author Contributions: B.L.: study conception and design, data collection, interpretation and analysis, drafting of the manuscript, critical revision for important intellectual content; P.-E.A.: data collection, interpretation and analysis, drafting of the manuscript; C.V.G.: data collection and interpretation, critical revision for important intellectual content; A.C.: study conception, critical revision for important intellectual content; J.H.: data collection and interpretation, critical revision for important intellectual content; A.S.: data collection and interpretation, critical revision for important intellectual content; M.S.: study conception and design, critical revision for important intellectual content; C.F.: study conception and design, critical revision for important intellectual content; S.T.: study conception and design, critical revision for important intellectual content; D.M.: study conception, critical revision for important intellectual content; F.P.: study conception and design, data collection, interpretation and analysis, drafting of the manuscript, critical revision for important intellectual content. All authors have read and agreed to the published version of the manuscript.

Funding: This research received no external funding.

Institutional Review Board Statement: The study was approved by the research ethics committee of Lille University Hospital.

Informed Consent Statement: Informed consent was obtained from all subjects involved in the study.

Data Availability Statement: The data presented in this study are available on reasonable request from the corresponding author, subject to approval by the research ethics committee of Lille University Hospital.

Conflicts of Interest: B.L.; P.-E.A.; C.V.G.; A.C.; J.H.; A.S.; D.M.; F.P. have no competing interest. They are employed by an institution engaged in a contractual collaboration with Siemens Healthineers. M.S.; C.F.; S.T. are employees of Siemens Healthineers.

References

1. Pennell, D.J.; Sechtem, U.P.; Higgins, C.B.; Manning, W.J.; Pohost, G.M.; Rademakers, F.E.; van Rossum, A.C.; Shaw, L.J.; Yucel, E.K.; Society for Cardiovascular Magnetic Resonance; et al. Clinical indications for cardiovascular magnetic resonance (CMR): Consensus Panel report. *Eur. Heart J.* **2004**, *25*, 1940–1965. [CrossRef] [PubMed]
2. Maceira, A.M.; Prasad, S.K.; Khan, M.; Pennell, D.J. Normalized left ventricular systolic and diastolic function by steady state free precession cardiovascular magnetic resonance. *J Cardiovasc. Magn. Reson.* **2006**, *8*, 417–426. [CrossRef]

3. Maceira, A.M.; Prasad, S.K.; Khan, M.; Pennell, D.J. Reference right ventricular systolic and diastolic function normalized to age, gender and body surface area from steady-state free precession cardiovascular magnetic resonance. *Eur. Heart J.* **2006**, *27*, 2879–2888. [CrossRef]
4. Grothues, F.; Moon, J.C.; Bellenger, N.G.; Smith, G.S.; Klein, H.U.; Pennell, D.J. Interstudy reproducibility of right ventricular volumes, function, and mass with cardiovascular magnetic resonance. *Am. Heart J.* **2004**, *147*, 218–223. [CrossRef]
5. Plein, S.; Bloomer, T.N.; Ridgway, J.P.; Jones, T.R.; Bainbridge, G.J.; Sivananthan, M.U. Steady-state free precession magnetic resonance imaging of the heart: Comparison with segmented k-space gradient-echo imaging. *J. Magn. Reson. Imaging* **2001**, *14*, 230–236. [CrossRef]
6. Lenz, G.W.; Haacke, E.M.; White, R.D. Retrospective cardiac gating: A review of technical aspects and future directions. *Magn. Reson. Imaging* **1989**, *7*, 445–455. [CrossRef]
7. Madore, B.; Hoge, W.S.; Chao, T.-C.; Zientara, G.P.; Chu, R. Retrospectively gated cardiac cine imaging with temporal and spatial acceleration. *Magn. Reson. Imaging* **2011**, *29*, 457–469. [CrossRef] [PubMed]
8. Nacif, M.S.; Zavodni, A.; Kawel, N.; Choi, E.-Y.; Lima, J.A.C.; Bluemke, D.A. Cardiac magnetic resonance imaging and its electrocardiographs (ECG): Tips and tricks. *Int. J. Cardiovasc. Imaging* **2012**, *28*, 1465–1475. [CrossRef]
9. Roussakis, A.; Baras, P.; Seimenis, I.; Andreou, J.; Danias, P.G. Relationship of number of phases per cardiac cycle and accuracy of measurement of left ventricular volumes, ejection fraction, and mass. *J. Cardiovasc. Magn. Reson. Off. J. Soc. Cardiovasc. Magn. Reson.* **2004**, *6*, 837–844. [CrossRef] [PubMed]
10. Miller, S.; Simonetti, O.P.; Carr, J.; Kramer, U.; Finn, J.P. MR imaging of the heart with cine true fast imaging with steady-state precession: Influence of spatial and temporal resolutions on left ventricular functional parameters. *Radiology* **2002**, *223*, 263–269. [CrossRef] [PubMed]
11. Donoho, D.L. Compressed sensing. *IEEE Trans. Inf. Theory* **2006**, *52*, 1289–1306. [CrossRef]
12. Candès, E.J.; Romberg, J.K.; Tao, T. Stable signal recovery from incomplete and inaccurate measurements. *Commun. Pure Appl. Math.* **2006**, *59*, 1207–1223. [CrossRef]
13. Lustig, M.; Donoho, D.; Pauly, J.M. Sparse MRI: The application of compressed sensing for rapid MR imaging. *Magn. Reson. Med.* **2007**, *58*, 1182–1195. [CrossRef] [PubMed]
14. Lustig, M.; Santos, J.M.; Lee, J.; Donoho, D.L.; Pauly, J.M. Application of compressed sensing for rapid MR imaging. In Proceedings of the 1st Signal Processing with Adaptive Sparse Structured Representations Workshop (SPARS 2005), Rennes, France, 16–18 November 2005; pp. 1–3.
15. Feng, L.; Srichai, M.B.; Lim, R.P.; Harrison, A.; King, W.; Adluru, G.; Dibella, E.V.R.; Sodickson, D.K.; Otazo, R.; Kim, D. Highly accelerated real-time cardiac cine MRI using k-t SPARSE-SENSE. *Magn. Reson. Med.* **2013**, *70*, 64–74. [CrossRef]
16. Vincenti, G.; Monney, P.; Chaptinel, J.; Rutz, T.; Coppo, S.; Zenge, M.O.; Schmidt, M.; Nadar, M.S.; Piccini, D.; Chèvre, P.; et al. Compressed sensing single-breath-hold CMR for fast quantification of LV function, volumes, and mass. *JACC Cardiovasc. Imaging* **2014**, *7*, 882–892. [CrossRef] [PubMed]
17. Goebel, J.; Nensa, F.; Schemuth, H.P.; Maderwald, S.; Gratz, M.; Quick, H.H.; Schlosser, T.; Nassenstein, K. Compressed sensing cine imaging with high spatial or high temporal resolution for analysis of left ventricular function. *J. Magn. Reson. Imaging* **2016**, *44*, 366–374. [CrossRef] [PubMed]
18. Haubenreisser, H.; Henzler, T.; Budjan, J.; Sudarski, S.; Zenge, M.O.; Schmidt, M.; Nadar, M.S.; Borggrefe, M.; Schoenberg, S.O.; Papavassiliu, T. Right ventricular imaging in 25 seconds: Evaluating the use of sparse sampling CINE with iterative reconstruction for volumetric analysis of the right ventricle. *Investig. Radiol.* **2016**, *51*, 379–386. [CrossRef]
19. Kido, T.; Kido, T.; Nakamura, M.; Watanabe, K.; Schmidt, M.; Forman, C.; Mochizuki, T. Compressed sensing real-time cine cardiovascular magnetic resonance: Accurate assessment of left ventricular function in a single-breath-hold. *J. Cardiovasc. Magn. Reson.* **2016**, *18*, 50–60. [CrossRef] [PubMed]
20. Vermersch, M.; Longère, B.; Coisne, A.; Schmidt, M.; Forman, C.; Monnet, A.; Pagniez, J.; Silvestri, V.; Simeone, A.; Cheasty, E.; et al. Compressed sensing real-time cine imaging for assessment of ventricular function, volumes and mass in clinical practice. *Eur. Radiol.* **2020**, *30*, 609–619. [CrossRef]
21. Goebel, J.; Nensa, F.; Schemuth, H.P.; Maderwald, S.; Quick, H.H.; Schlosser, T.; Nassenstein, K. Real-Time SPARSE-SENSE cine MR imaging in atrial fibrillation: A feasibility study. *Acta Radiol.* **2017**, *58*, 922–928. [CrossRef]
22. Klinke, V.; Muzzarelli, S.; Lauriers, N.; Locca, D.; Vincenti, G.; Monney, P.; Lu, C.; Nothnagel, D.; Pilz, G.; Lombardi, M.; et al. Quality assessment of cardiovascular magnetic resonance in the setting of the European CMR registry: Description and validation of standardized criteria. *J. Cardiovasc. Magn. Reson.* **2013**, *15*, 55. [CrossRef]
23. Larson, A.C.; Kellman, P.; Arai, A.; Hirsch, G.A.; McVeigh, E.; Li, D.; Simonetti, O.P. Preliminary investigation of respiratory self-gating for free-breathing segmented cine MRI. *Magn. Reson. Med.* **2005**, *53*, 159–168. [CrossRef]
24. Wetzl, J.; Schmidt, M.; Pontana, F.; Longère, B.; Lugauer, F.; Maier, A.; Hornegger, J.; Forman, C. Single-breath-hold 3-D CINE imaging of the left ventricle using cartesian sampling. *Magn. Reson. Mater. Phys. Biol. Med.* **2017**, *31*, 19–31. [CrossRef]
25. Richard, S.; Husarik, D.B.; Yadava, G.; Murphy, S.N.; Samei, E. Towards task-based assessment of CT performance: System and object MTF across different reconstruction algorithms. *Med. Phys.* **2012**, *39*, 4115–4122. [CrossRef] [PubMed]
26. Benchoufi, M.; Matzner-Lober, E.; Molinari, N.; Jannot, A.-S.; Soyer, P. Interobserver agreement issues in radiology. *Diagn. Interv. Imaging* **2020**, *101*, 639–641. [CrossRef]
27. Graff, C.G.; Sidky, E.Y. Compressive sensing in medical imaging. *Appl. Opt.* **2015**, *54*, C23–C44. [CrossRef] [PubMed]

28. Li, T.; Feng, H.; Xu, Z. A New analytical edge spread function fitting model for modulation transfer function measurement. *Chin. Opt. Lett.* **2011**, *9*, 031101. [CrossRef]
29. Lurz, P.; Muthurangu, V.; Schievano, S.; Nordmeyer, J.; Bonhoeffer, P.; Taylor, A.M.; Hansen, M.S. Feasibility and reproducibility of biventricular volumetric assessment of cardiac function during exercise using real-time radial k-t SENSE magnetic resonance imaging. *J. Magn. Reson. Imaging JMRI* **2009**, *29*, 1062–1070. [CrossRef] [PubMed]
30. Voit, D.; Zhang, S.; Unterberg-Buchwald, C.; Sohns, J.M.; Lotz, J.; Frahm, J. Real-time cardiovascular magnetic resonance at 1.5 T using balanced SSFP and 40 ms resolution. *J. Cardiovasc. Magn. Reson. Off. J. Soc. Cardiovasc. Magn. Reson.* **2013**, *15*, 79–86. [CrossRef] [PubMed]
31. Zhang, S.; Uecker, M.; Voit, D.; Merboldt, K.-D.; Frahm, J. Real-time cardiovascular magnetic resonance at high temporal resolution: Radial FLASH with nonlinear inverse reconstruction. *J. Cardiovasc. Magn. Reson. Off. J. Soc. Cardiovasc. Magn. Reson.* **2010**, *12*, 39–45. [CrossRef] [PubMed]
32. Fraden, J. *Handbook of Modern Sensors—Physics, Designs and Applications*, 3rd ed.; Springer: New York, NY, USA, 2004.

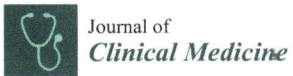

Article

Impact of Morphotype on Image Quality and Diagnostic Performance of Ultra-Low-Dose Chest CT

Anne-Claire Ortlieb [1], Aissam Labani [2], François Severac [3], Mi-Young Jeung [2], Catherine Roy [2] and Mickaël Ohana [2,4,*]

[1] Radiology Department, Institut Paoli-Calmettes, 232 Boulevard de Sainte-Marguerite, 13009 Marseille, France; anneclaireor@gmail.com
[2] Radiology Department, Nouvel Hôpital Civil, 1 Place de l'Hôpital, 67000 Strasbourg, France; aissam.labani@chru-strasbourg.fr (A.L.); Mi-Young.Jeung@chru-strasbourg.fr (M.-Y.J.); catherine.roy@chru-strasbourg.fr (C.R.)
[3] Biostatistics Department, Nouvel Hôpital Civil, 1 Place de l'Hôpital, 67000 Strasbourg, France francois.severac@chru-strasbourg.fr
[4] ICube Laboratory, 300 Boulevard Sébastien Brandt, 67200 Illkirch Graffenstaden, France
* Correspondence: mickael.ohana@chru-strasbourg.fr

Citation: Ortlieb, A.-C.; Labani, A.; Severac, F.; Jeung, M.-Y.; Roy, C.; Ohana, M. Impact of Morphotype on Image Quality and Diagnostic Performance of Ultra-Low-Dose Chest CT. *J. Clin. Med.* **2021**, *10*, 3284. https://doi.org/10.3390/jcm10153284

Academic Editor: Ernesto Di Cesare

Received: 16 June 2021
Accepted: 22 July 2021
Published: 26 July 2021

Publisher's Note: MDPI stays neutral with regard to jurisdictional claims in published maps and institutional affiliations.

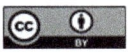

Copyright: © 2021 by the authors. Licensee MDPI, Basel, Switzerland. This article is an open access article distributed under the terms and conditions of the Creative Commons Attribution (CC BY) license (https://creativecommons.org/licenses/by/4.0/).

Abstract: Objectives: The image quality of an Ultra-Low-Dose (ULD) chest CT depends on the patient's morphotype. We hypothesize that there is a threshold beyond which the diagnostic performance of a ULD chest CT is too degraded. This work assesses the influence of morphotype (Body Mass Index BMI, Maximum Transverse Chest Diameter MTCD and gender) on image quality and the diagnostic performance of a ULD chest CT. Methods: A total of 170 patients from three prior prospective monocentric studies were retrospectively included. Renewal of consent was waived by our IRB. All the patients underwent two consecutive unenhanced chest CT acquisitions with a full dose (120 kV, automated tube current modulation) and a ULD (135 kV, fixed tube current at 10 mA). Image noise, subjective image quality and diagnostic performance for nine predefined lung parenchyma lesions were assessed by two independent readers, and correlations with the patient's morphotype were sought. Results: The mean BMI was 26.6 ± 5.3; 20.6% of patients had a BMI > 30. There was a statistically significant negative correlation of the BMI with the image quality ($\rho = -0.32$; IC95% = (−0.468; −0.18)). The per-patient diagnostic performance of ULD was sensitivity, 77%; specificity, 99%; PPV, 94% and NPV, 65%. There was no statistically significant influence of the BMI, the MTCD nor the gender on the per-patient and per-lesion diagnostic performance of a ULD chest CT, apart from a significant negative correlation for the detection of emphysema. Conclusions: Despite a negative correlation between the BMI and the image quality of a ULD chest CT, we did not find a correlation between the BMI and the diagnostic performance of the examination, suggesting a possible use of the ULD protocol in obese patients.

Keywords: multidetector computed tomography; radiation dosage; lung; helical computed tomography

1. Introduction

Computed Tomography (CT) accounts for the large majority of medical exposures to ionizing radiation [1]. In chest imaging, the radiation dose delivered varies significantly between clinical indications, machine and institution [2] and the dose-length product (DLP) is estimated at 347 mGy·cm (50th percentile) in a 2017 review of 159,909 US patients [3]. Significant susceptible organs such as the breasts, lungs and thyroid are included in the field-of-view; this justifies the reduction in the radiation dose delivered to the minimum needed for adequate diagnosis [4,5].

Chest CT is an appropriate candidate to a significant radiation dose reduction, due to an overall low attenuation of the lung parenchyma resulting in a high contrast. Substantial efforts have been made to optimize the dose delivered in chest imaging, particularly through the implementation of iterative reconstruction [6] and deep learning reconstruction techniques [7]. It is now possible to achieve a diagnostic chest CT at the radiation dose of a posteroanterior and lateral chest radiograph series [8,9], and this has been proven efficient for various clinical scenarios [10], such as lung nodule detection and follow-up [11,12], pulmonary infection [13], CT-guided percutaneous biopsy [14], lymphangioleiomyomatosis [15], etc. However, the image quality of these Ultra-Low-Dose (ULD) chest CTs remains dependent on the patient's morphotype, and prior studies [11,16] seldomly included patients with a Body Mass Index (BMI) greater than 30 kg·m^{-2}. Consequently, the diagnostic performance of a ULD chest CT is not well documented in obese patients [17].

We hypothesize that beyond a certain morphotype, defined by a threshold of BMI and/or a threshold of Maximum Transverse Chest Diameter (MTCD) and/or gender (given the different distribution of fat and breasts between women and men), the deterioration of the image quality becomes too important and leads to a decrease in the diagnostic performance.

The objective of this study was, therefore, to determine the influence of these morphological parameters (BMI, MTCD and gender) on the objective and subjective image quality of a ULD chest CT and on its diagnostic performance for the detection of nine predefined pulmonary parenchymal lesions.

2. Materials and Methods

2.1. Population

All 170 patients from 3 prior prospective studies performed in Strasbourg University Hospital and carried out on the same second-generation 320-row scanner (Aquillion One Vision Edition, Toshiba, Japan), were retrospectively included. The first study [18] included 55 patients from July 2013 to May 2014 with an occupational exposure to asbestos of at least 15 years, referred for screening of asbestos-related pleuro-pulmonary lesions. The second study [19] (April 2014 to September 2014) and the third study [20] (April 2015 to September 2015) included 51 and 64 patients, respectively, that were referred for a clinically indicated unenhanced chest CT.

The inclusion criterion common to the 3 studies was an age greater or equal to 35 years for men and 40 years for women. The common exclusion criteria were pregnancy, the inability to maintain apnea for more than 5 s, the inability to raise the arms above the head and the inability to give informed consent.

The renewal of consent was not required for this retrospective study by our hospital institutional review board. Written informed consent and approval from the local Ethics Committee had been obtained in the first instance for all patients, at the time of their initial prospective inclusion in one of the 3 trials.

Age, gender, weight, height, BMI and clinical indication for chest CT were recorded at the time of the examination. The Maximum Transverse Chest Diameter (MTCD) was measured by a radiologist (AC, with 4 years of experience in chest CT) on a mediastinal window, from lateral thoracic wall to lateral thoracic wall.

2.2. CT Acquisition

Each patient underwent an unenhanced chest CT with two successive acquisitions: one "full dose" (FD) acquisition (120 kV, automated tube current modulation maxed at 700 mA) used as the Gold Standard and one "Ultra-Low-Dose" (ULD) acquisition (135 kV, 10 mA fixed) [21]. Acquisitions were made on a second-generation 320-row scanner (Aquillion One Vision Edition, Canon), with the parameters given in Table 1. All examinations were performed in successive end-inspiratory apneas, arms raised above the head. The 55 patients from the first study were acquired in prone position, to avoid gravity-dependent posterior parenchymal abnormalities—as recommended when screening for asbestos-related diseases [18]. The 115 patients from the two following studies were acquired in supine position. The posterior–anterior and lateral topograms were used to define the acquisition field, extending from the pulmonary apexes to the diaphragm; the acquisition length was kept identical for the two consecutive FD and ULD acquisitions.

Table 1. Acquisition parameters of study protocols.

	ULD-CT	FD-CT (Reference)
Voltage (kV)	135	120
Tube current (mA)	10	80–700
Tube current-time product (mAs)	3	20–200
Pitch	0.813	0.813
Rotation time (s)	0.275	0.275
Collimation	0.5 × 80	0.5 × 80
Reconstructed slice thickness (mm)	1	-
Reconstruction algorithm	AIDR-3D	AIDR-3D

The FD and ULD acquisitions were reconstructed in lung window (width = 1500 HU; center = −700 HU) with a hard kernel and a slice thickness of 1 mm, using the constructor's iterative reconstruction algorithm set at a standard level (Adaptative Iterative Dose Reduction using 3 Dimensional AIDR-3D, Canon).

The whole set of 340 parenchymal reconstructions were anonymized and randomized into two series of 170 FD and 170 ULD examinations, in a different random order for both.

2.3. Dosimetry

Radiation doses were expressed in dose-length product (DLP). The effective radiation dose (ED) was calculated by multiplying the DLP by the chest-specific conversion factor of 0.014 mSv/mGy·cm [22].

2.4. Quantitative Image Quality

Image noise was defined as the standard deviation (SD) of the attenuation of air within the tracheal lumen, using a circular region of interest (ROI) averaging at least 40 mm^2, 1 cm above the carina, in the parenchymal reconstruction. It was measured three times by the same reader (AC), with size and position of the ROI kept constant between patients. The average of the three measurements was used as the final value in the statistical analysis.

2.5. Qualitative Image Quality

The overall subjective image quality of ULD acquisitions was assessed independently by two radiologists that specialized in chest imaging (M.O., with 9 years of experience in chest CT and A.C., with 4 years of experience) using a 5-point Likert scale (Table 2), after a training session with joint evaluation of 15 cases.

Table 2. Subjective image quality for ULD chest CT.

	Subjective Image Quality	Ratings
1	Unacceptable image quality	*non-diagnostic examination*
2	Poor image quality	
3	Moderate image quality	*diagnostic examination*
4	Good image quality	
5	Excellent image quality	

2.6. Diagnostic Performance

Each radiologist independently read the ULD then the FD lung parenchyma acquisitions, both in a different random order and with a delay of at least two weeks in between to limit the risk of a memorization bias.

All images were analyzed on a dedicated Workstation (Vitrea version 6.4, Vital Images), with use of multiplanar reconstructions and Maximum Intensity Projection. For each acquisition, the presence or absence of 9 predefined parenchymal lesions, based on the Fleischner Society lexicon [23] was rated in a binary fashion (i.e., presence or absence of the anomaly). The following lesions were assessed: solid nodule ≥ 5 mm, ground glass nodule, mass ≥ 3 cm, ground glass opacity, alveolar consolidation, emphysema, interlobular septal thickening, bronchiectasis, fibrosis.

Disagreements between readers were resolved in a subsequent consensual reading session. The consensual analysis of the FD chest CT served as the reference standard to which the consensual analysis of ULD CT was compared.

2.7. Statistical Analysis

Quantitative variables were reported as average ± SD or median (1st quartile; 3rd quartile) according to their Gaussian distribution and assessed using the Shapiro–Wilk test. Categorical variables were reported as frequencies or percentages.

The inter-reader agreement for the subjective assessment of image quality was determined using Cohen's kappa and quadratic weighting to account for the degree of disagreement. The confidence intervals for Cohen's Kappa coefficients were calculated using the Bootstrap method. A kappa value of (0.0–0.20] was regarded as poor, (0.2–0.40] as fair, (0.41–0.60] as moderate, (0.61–0.80] as good and (0.81–1.00] as excellent.

Continuous variables were compared with a Student's t-test when the parametric conditions were met, and otherwise with a Wilcoxon test.

The Pearson χ^2 test or the Fisher exact test were used to compare the effectiveness of lesion detection (presence or absence) among the two groups, based on theoretical numbers.

Correlations between continuous variables were evaluated using the Spearman's correlation coefficient. Comparison between the different correlation coefficients were made using the Hotelling Williams test.

Diagnostic performance of the ULD chest CT for the detection of 9 pulmonary lesions was compared to the FD chest CT: the sensitivity (Se), specificity (Sp), positive predictive value (PPV), negative predictive value (NPV), accuracy and error rate were calculated using a confidence interval of 95%.

A p-value smaller than 0.05 was considered statistically significant.

All statistical analyses were performed using R software, version 3.4.3. R Core Team (2015). (R: *A language and environment for statistical computing*. R Foundation for Statistical Computing).

3. Results

3.1. Population

A total of 170 patients were retrospectively included: 129 men (75.9%) and 41 women (24.1%). Age was 62.7 ± 11 years old (range 35–88).

The clinical indications were screening of asbestos-related pleuro-pulmonary diseases ($n = 55$), follow-up of pulmonary nodules ($n = 39$), pulmonary infections ($n = 23$), follow-up of lung cancer ($n = 13$), follow-up of interstitial pulmonary diseases ($n = 10$), follow-up of chronic obstructive lung diseases ($n = 4$) and other situations ($n = 26$).

The mean BMI was 26.6 ± 5.3 kg·m^{-2} (range 14.5–54.9), with a median BMI of 25.8 kg·m^{-2} (IQ 23.1–29.3). Of the patients, 45.9% ($n = 78$) had a BMI less than or equal to 25 kg·m^{-2}; 33.5% ($n = 57$) had a BMI between 25 and 30 kg·m^{-2} and 20.6% ($n = 35$) had a BMI greater than or equal to 30 kg·m^{-2}, of which eight patients (4.7% of the population) had a BMI greater than 35 kg·m^{-2}.

The MTCD was 35.5 ± 3.4 cm (range 27–46).

3.2. Dosimetry

The DLP for FD acquisitions was 252.4 ± 143.2 mGy·cm (range 84.2–868.5), with a median of 204.4 mGy·cm (IQ 152.9–323.2). The average ED was estimated at 3.46 mSv.

The DLP for ULD acquisitions was 16.4 ± 1.8 mGy·cm (12.1–20.8), with a median of 16.3 mGy·cm (IQ 15.4–17.7). The average ED was estimated at 0.23 mSv, representing a 93% decrease compared to the FD acquisition.

3.3. Quantitative Image Quality

Image noise was 39.9 ± 11.3 for FD acquisitions and 53.3 ± 14.1 for ULD acquisitions, corresponding to a 33% increase.

There was no statistically significant correlation between BMI and noise in the ULD acquisitions: $\rho = -0.12$; 95% CI (-0.263–0.015); $p = 0.11$ (Figure 1).

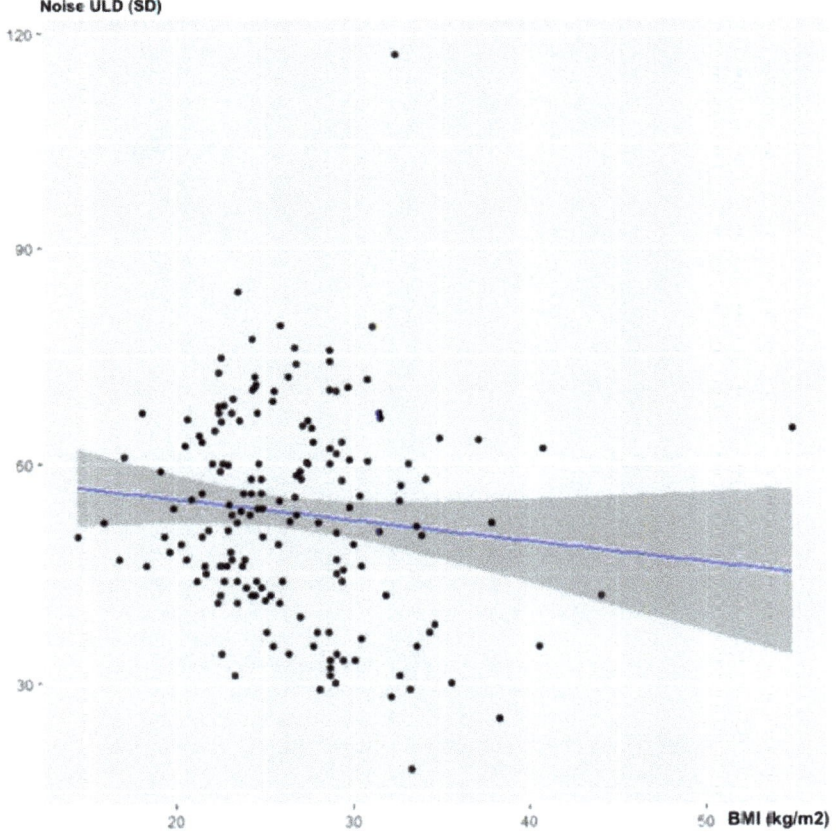

Figure 1. Influence of BMI on noise for ULD-CT.

There was no statistically significant correlation between MTCD and noise in the ULD acquisitions: $\rho = -0.14$; 95% CI (-0.276–0.007); $p = 0.07$ (Figure 2).

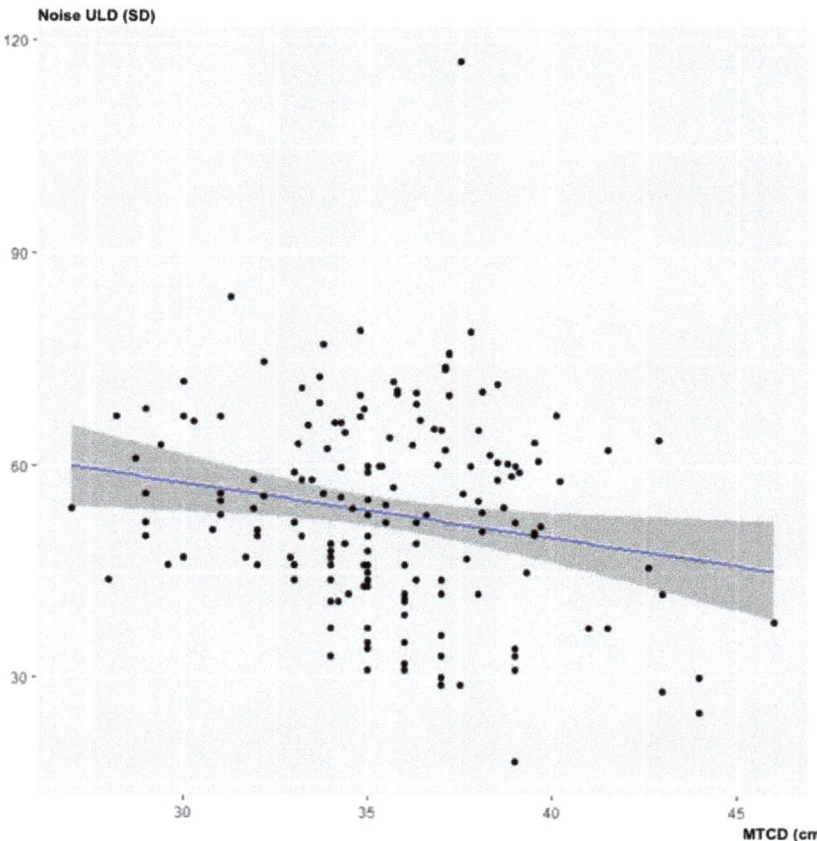

Figure 2. Influence of MTCD on image noise (in SD) for ULD-CT.

3.4. Subjective Image Quality

The inter-reader agreement for the overall subjective image quality score was good, with a Cohen's Kappa of 0.61 (95% CI [0.46–0.72]; $p < 0.001$). The average score assigned by the two readers for ULD image quality was ultimately 4.5 ± 0.6 with a median of 5 (4.5–5). The overall subjective image quality was almost always diagnostic (i.e., equal to or greater than three), except for two patients according to the junior reader (BMI at 44.1 and 37.8 kg·m^{-2}) and one patient according to the senior reader (BMI at 44.1 kg·m^{-2}). The distribution of the ratings is detailed in Table 3. An illustrative example is given in Figure 3.

Table 3. Distribution of ratings for subjective image quality.

Notes	R1	R2	Average
1	0 (0%)	0 (0%)	0
2	2 (1.2%)	1 (0.6%)	1.5
3	10 (5.9%)	19 (11.2%)	14.5
4	38 (22.3%)	51 (30%)	44.5
5	120 (70.6%)	99 (58.2%)	109.5
Average ± SD	4.62 ± 0.65	4.46 ± 0.71	4.5 ± 0.70

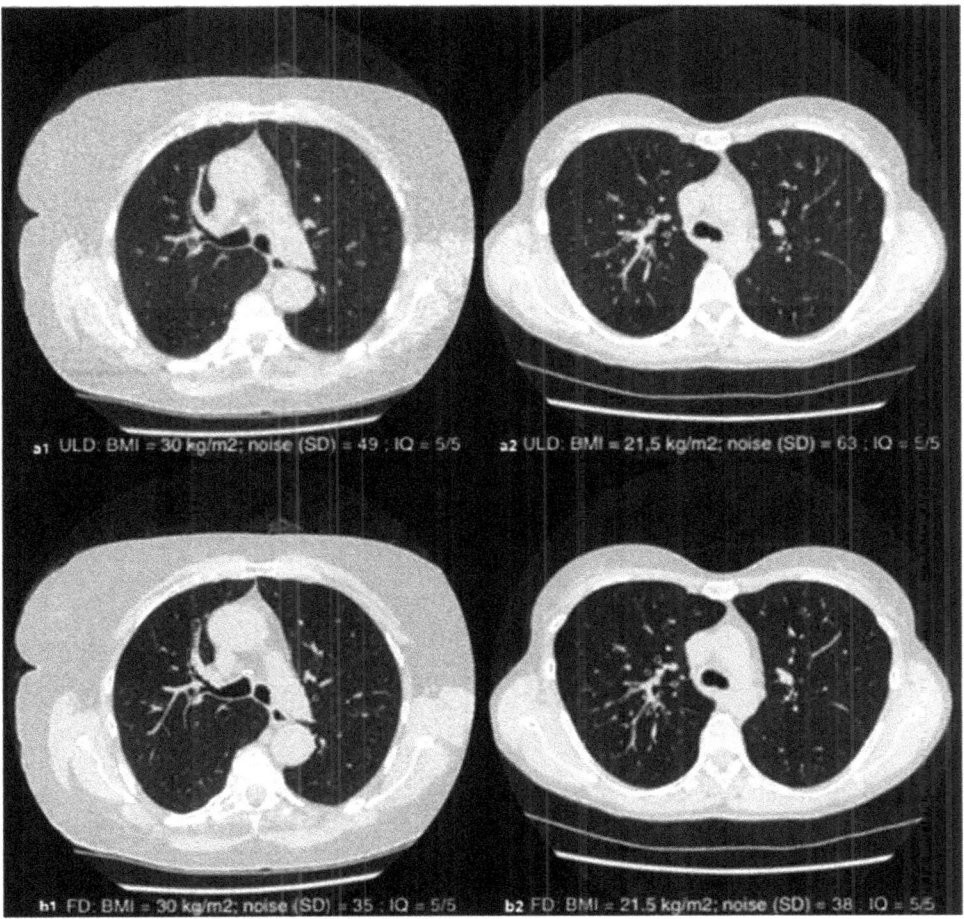

Figure 3. Axial slices in parenchymal window illustrating the subjective quality of the ULD (**a1,a2**) and FD (**b1,b2**) acquisitions in patients with a BMI of 30 kg·m^{-2} (1) and 21.5 kg·m^{-2} (2): diagnostic-quality images (QI = 5/5) despite the different morphotype.

The BMI was negatively and significantly correlated with the subjective image quality of the ULD acquisitions, with a correlation coefficient of $\rho = -0.325$; 95% CI (-0.462; -0.178); $p < 0.001$ (Figure 4).

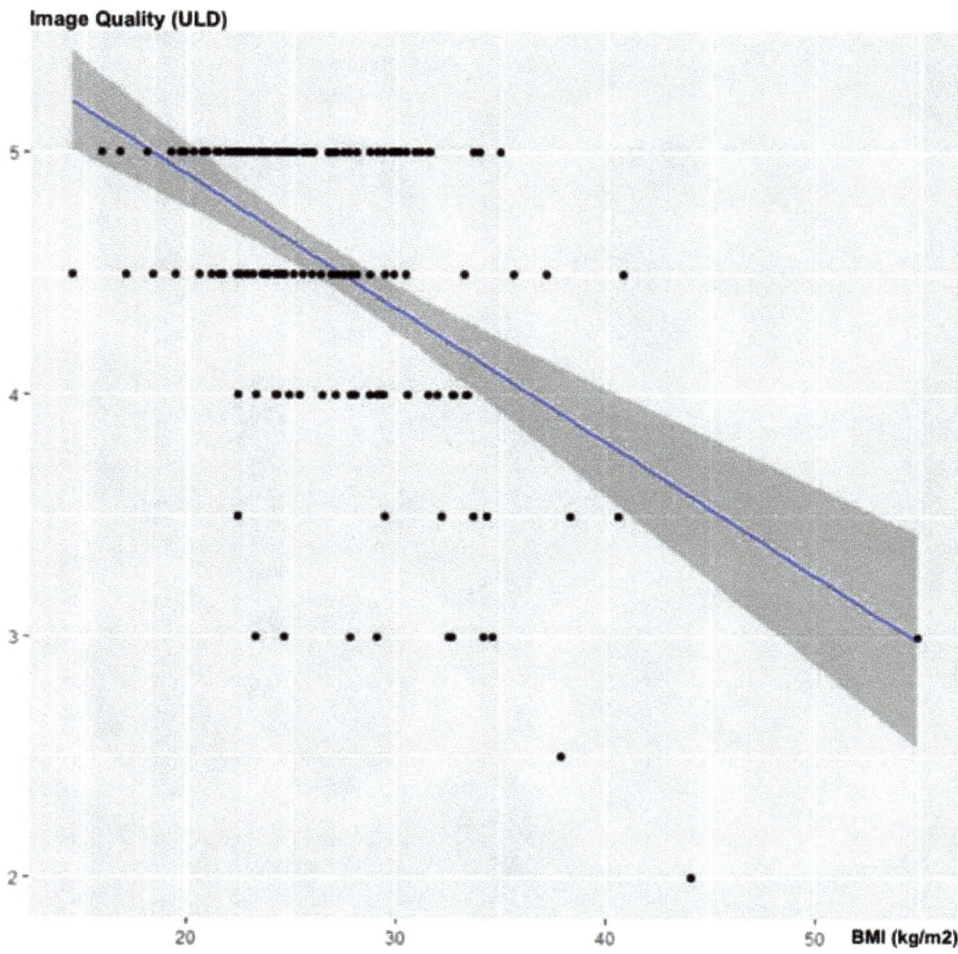

Figure 4. Influence of the BMI on subjective image quality.

There was no statistically significant correlation between the MTCD and the subjective image quality of the ULD acquisitions: $\rho = -0.0979$; 95% CI $(-0.253–0.055)$; $p = 0.2041$ (Figure 5).

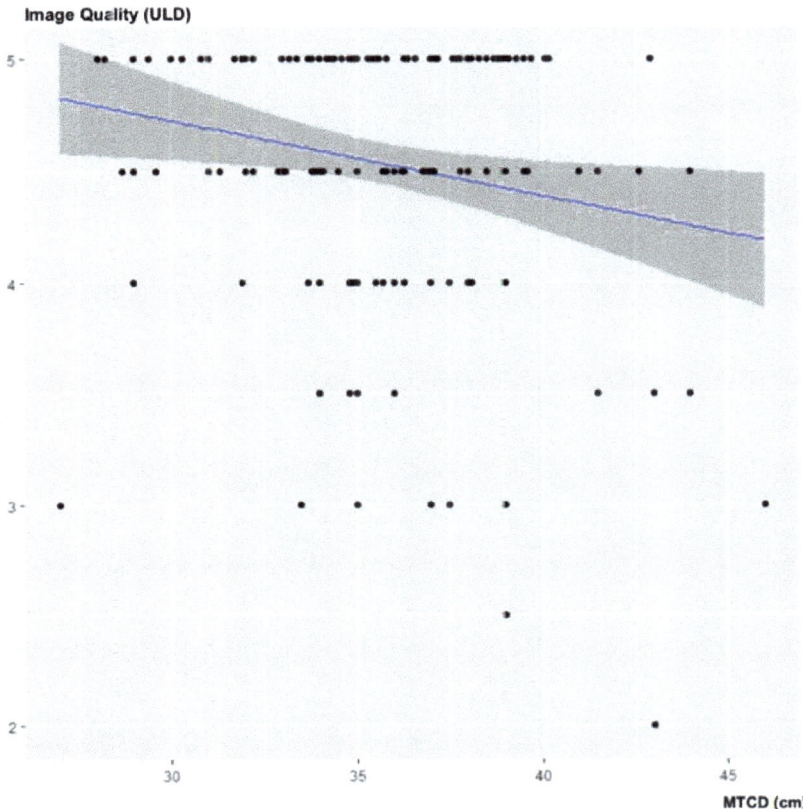

Figure 5. Influence of the MTCD on subjective image quality.

3.5. Diagnostic Performance

At least one predefined parenchymal lesion was found in 114 (67%) out of the 170 examinations, with a total of 243 lesions on the reference FD acquisition. There was a disagreement in the reading of the reference CT scan in 44 patients: non-agreement rate = 25.9%; 95% CI, (19.5–33.2].

3.6. Diagnostic Performance per Patient

The overall diagnostic performance of the ULD chest CT (all lesions considered) were sensitivity, 77%; specificity, 99%; PPV, 94% and NPV, 65%.

The overall agreement rate for the interpretation of the ULD-CT scanner for all the lesions considered (disagreement = at least one difference out of nine lesions), was 68% (116/170; 95% CI [60.67–75.15].

There was no statistically significant correlation between BMI ($p = 0.34$), MTCD ($p = 0.92$) or gender ($p = 0.53$) and the per-patient diagnostic performance of the ULD-CT.

3.7. Diagnostic Performance per Lesion

The diagnostic performances per lesion are summarized in Table 4.

Table 4. Diagnostic performance of ULD-CT.

	Number of Lesions (n)	ULD-CT vs. FD-CT				Error Rate %
		Se (%)	Sp (%)	VPP (%)	VPN (%)	
Abnormalities	243	77 (188/243)	99 (1276/1287)	94 (188/199)	65 (860/1331)	25.9
Solid nodule	66	86 (57/66)	94 (98/104)	90 (57/63)	92 (98/107)	9
95% CI		[0.75; 0.93]	[0.88; 0.98]	[0.80; 0.96]	[0.84; 0.96]	
Ground glass nodule	8	62 (5/8)	99 (161/162)	83 (5/6)	98 (161/164)	2
95% CI		[0.24; 0.91]	[0.97; 0.99]	[0.36; 0.99]	[0.95; 0.99]	
Mass > 3 cm	3	100 (3/3)	100 (167/167)	100 (3/3)	100 (167/167)	0
95% CI		[0.29; 1]	[0.98; 1]	[0.29; 1]	0.98; 1]	
Ground glass opacity	30	70 (21/30)	99 (139/140)	95 (21/22)	94 (139/148)	6
95% CI		[0.51; 0.85]	[0.96; 0.99]	[0.77; 0.99]	[0.89; 0.97]	
Alveolar consolidation	24	83 (20/24)	99 (144/146)	91 (20/22)	97 (144/148)	4
95% CI		[0.63; 0.95]	[0.95; 0.99]	[0.71; 0.99]	0.93; 0.99]	
Emphysema	58	81 (47/58)	99 (111/112)	98 (47/48)	91 (111/122)	7
95% CI		[0.69; 0.90]	[0.95; 0.99]	[0.89; 0.99]	[0.84; 0.95]	
Interstitial septal thickening	11	45 (5/11)	100 (159/159)	100 (5/5)	96 (159/165)	4
95% CI		[0.17; 0.77]	[0.98; 1]	[0.48; 1]	[0.92; 0.99]	
Bronchiectasis	31	71 (22/31)	100 (139/139)	100 (22/22)	94 (139/148)	5
95% CI		[0.52; 0.86]	[0.97; 1]	[0.85; 1]	[0.89; 0.97]	
Fibrosis	12	67 (8/12)	100 (158/158)	100 (8/8)	98 (158/162)	2
95% CI		[0.35; 0.90]	[0.98; 1]	[0.63; 1]	[0.94; 0.99]	

There was a statistically significant negative influence of the BMI on the diagnostic performance of the ULD CT for the detection of emphysema ($p < 0.001$). This negative correlation was not statistically found for the MTCD nor the gender.

There was no statistically significant correlation between BMI, MTCD or gender and the diagnostic performances for the eight other parenchymal lesions, provided that some lesions had a low incidence (ground glass nodules, masses, alveolar consolidation, septal thickening and fibrosis).

4. Discussion

Our study compiling 170 patients found an overall sensitivity of 77%, specificity of 99% and an agreement rate of 74.1% for a ULD chest CT when compared to the reference FD CT, using standard iterative reconstruction techniques. Despite the statistically significant negative correlation between image quality and BMI ($\rho = -0.325$; $p < 0.001$), we did not find a negative correlation between BMI and diagnostic performance (per patients or per lesions, except for emphysema). As a result, the deterioration in the image quality of a ULD CT associated with the increase in BMI does not translate into a significant decrease in diagnostic performance. Based on these findings, we can recommend the use of ULD CT, even when the BMI is greater than 30 kg·m^{-2}, and likely up to 35 kg·m^2 based on the BMI distribution in our population.

In prior publications, most studies did not include patients with a BMI greater than 30 kg·m^{-2}.

In his study, Lee [11] compared the ULD CT (80 kV-30 mA fixed) to a low-dose (LD) CT in 81 patients, the average BMI of the population was 23.6 ± 3.8 kg·m^{-2} and only four patients had a BMI greater than 30 kg·m^{-2}. They demonstrated a significant influence of

BMI on the subjective image quality of the ULD CT ($\rho = -0.480$; $p < 0.001$), with the images being of diagnostic-quality in more than 95% of cases when the BMI was lower than 25, compared to only 70% when the BMI was greater than 25.

In the publication of a study conducted by Kim [13] using ULD CT (120 kV-15 mA fixed) in patients with neutropenic fever, all of the 207 patients included had a BMI lower than 30 kg·m^{-2} and only 14% of them had a BMI greater than 25 kg·m^{-2}, among them four had a non-diagnostic image quality.

In Macri et al.'s study [16], using 100 kV and automated tube current modulation (60 mAs reference), a large majority of the patients included had a normal BMI (average BMI of 23.9 kg·m^{-2} for men and 23.1 kg·m^{-2} for women) and the image quality was excellent for 90% of the patients with a BMI up to 25, compared to only 76% of patients with a BMI greater than 25. It showed an excellent agreement between the ULD-CT results compared to LD-CT, except in two patients with a BMI at 26.8 and 27.4 kg·m^{-2}.

Messerli et al. [12] studied the diagnostic performance of a ULD chest CT (100 kV, fixed tube current at 70 mAs, tin filtration) on the detection of pulmonary nodule compared to the reference FD CT. The population studied included 202 patients with a mean BMI of 26.2 ± 5.3 kg·m^{-2} (range 15.9–49), and the results showed a significantly decreased subjective image quality for the ULD CT in patients with a BMI greater than 30 ($p < 0.001$), in line with our findings. However, the number of patients with a BMI greater than 30 was not specified in the article. The authors found a statistically significant negative influence of the BMI on the sensitivity of the ULD-CT for the detection of pulmonary nodules: the sensitivity for the detection of all nodules was 92.6% in patients with a BMI of 25 compared to 84.9% in patients with a BMI of 35, which differs with our results.

To summarize, previous studies seldomly included obese patients (BMI > 30 kg·m^{-2}) and always reported a significant deterioration in image quality for high BMI. Only nodules were analyzed, and conclusions were in favor of a negative correlation between diagnostic performance and BMI. Our work, which includes a significantly higher number of obese patients (35 patients) nuance these observations by confirming a negative correlation between subjective image quality and BMI, yet without negatively impacting the diagnostic performance for the detection of nodules and seven other parenchymal lesions.

There was no statistically significant correlation between the MTCD and the subjective image quality, confirming BMI as the only metric that can predict the image quality expected from a ULD CT examination. This is all the more useful since BMI is easily obtained before the acquisition. BMI and MTCD had an unexpected—even though not significant—tendency to lower the image noise. This positive influence could be explained by the high capacity of iterative reconstruction methods to significantly reduce noise. Similar results can be extracted from the literature [24,25], where images reconstructed with ASIR were associated with a greater noise reduction in high-weight patients.

The diagnostic performance of the ULD-CT was lower for emphysema and ground glass nodule compared to solid nodule and alveolar consolidation, which is in line with previous publications that have shown excellent diagnostic performance for spontaneously high contrast pulmonary lesions and lower performance for less attenuating lesions [11]. Unlike in the studies by Lee [11] and Macri [16], we chose to compare the diagnostic performance of the ULD CT to a reference "full dose" CT, which is the current Gold standard.

Several limitations of this work must be mentioned.

First, its retrospective nature—even if it is based on three prospective studies—and the relatively small number of severely obese patients (BMI > 35 kg·m^{-2})—even if this number is higher than in all the other publications on the subject.

Second, the population included in our study was mainly male, this is probably due to an inclusion bias for the 55 patients from the study that analyzed asbestos-related diseases and included only men. Nevertheless, the statistical analysis did not reveal any significant correlation by gender. Indeed, with breast attenuation being more significant in women, one could have imagined that at an equal BMI, the female sex could negatively influence the subjective image quality of the ULD CT.

Third, one third of the population was acquired in the prone position, which might have an impact on image quality.

Fourth, as a limitation inherent to all in vivo studies, reference was based only on the consensual reading of the FD CT by two readers, with a lack of any pathological confirmation. In the evaluation of subtle parenchymal lesions such as ground glass opacities, the analysis of multiple reviewers with different levels of expertise might have been more appropriate, as it could have led to a stronger consensus.

Finally, one should mention the monovendor nature of this study, carried out with a unique ULD acquisition protocol with a fixed tube current and a single iterative reconstruction algorithm. The prior publications listed used different iterative reconstruction software, and although our results are comparable to those studies, they cannot be strictly generalized to other constructors and other reconstruction techniques. Of note, the recently introduced Deep Learning Reconstruction might well further enhance the robustness of low dose acquisitions to high BMIs [26].

To conclude, our study suggests that despite a significant negative correlation of the BMI with the image quality of a ULD chest CT, its diagnostic performance is maintained. Consequently, the use of a ULD protocol when an unenhanced chest CT is needed could remain relevant in patients with a BMI greater than 30 kg·m^{-2}.

Author Contributions: Conceptualization, M.O.; methodology, F.S.; validation, M.O. and C.R.; formal analysis, F.S. and A.-C.O.; investigation, A.-C.O., M.O. and A.L.; resources, A.L., C.R. and M.-Y.J.; data curation, A.-C.O. and M.O.; writing—original draft preparation, A.-C.O.; writing—review and editing, M.O.; visualization, A.-C.O., A.L., F.S., M.-Y.J., C.R. and M.O.; supervision, C.R. and M.O.; project administration, C.R. All authors have read and agreed to the published version of the manuscript.

Funding: This research received no external funding.

Institutional Review Board Statement: The renewal of consent was not required for this retrospective study by our hospital institutional review board.

Informed Consent Statement: Written informed consent and approval from the local Ethics Committee had been obtained in the first instance for all patients, at the time of their initial prospective inclusion in one of the three trials.

Conflicts of Interest: The authors declare no conflict of interest.

Abbreviations

BMI	Body Mass Index
CT	Computed Tomography
DLP	Dose length Product
ED	Effective Dose
FD	Full Dose
MTCD	Maximum Transverse Chest Diameter
ROI	Region Of Interest
SD	Standard Deviation
ULD	Ultra-Low Dose

References

1. Brenner, D.J.; Hall, E.J. Computed Tomography—An Increasing Source of Radiation Exposure. *N. Engl. J. Med.* **2007**, *357*, 2277–2284. [CrossRef]
2. Ohana, M.; Ludes, C.; Schaal, M.; Meyer, E.; Jeung, M.-Y.; Labani, A.; Roy, C. Quel avenir pour la radiographie thoracique face au scanner ultra-low dose? *Rev. Pneumol. Clin.* **2017**, *73*, 3–12. [CrossRef] [PubMed]
3. Kanal, K.M.; Butler, P.F.; Sengupta, D.; Bhargavan-Chatfield, M.; Coombs, L.P.; Morin, R.L. U.S. Diagnostic Reference Levels and Achievable Doses for 10 Adult CT Examinations. *Radiology* **2017**, *284*, 120–133. [CrossRef]

4. Sarma, A.; Heilbrun, M.E.; Conner, K.E.; Stevens, S.M.; Woller, S.C.; Elliott, C.G. Radiation and Chest CT Scan Examinations. *Chest* **2012**, *142*, 750–760. [CrossRef] [PubMed]
5. Nicolan, B.; Greffier, J.; Dabli, D.; de Forges, H.; Arcis, E.; Al Zouabi, N.; Larbi, A.; Beregi, J.-P.; Frandon, J. Diagnostic performance of ultra-low dose versus standard dose CT for non-traumatic abdominal emergencies. *Diagn. Interv. Imaging* **2021**, *102*, 379–387. [CrossRef] [PubMed]
6. Beister, M.; Kolditz, D.; Kalender, W.A. Iterative reconstruction methods in X-ray CT. *Phys. Med.* **2012**, *28*, 94–108. [CrossRef]
7. Singh, R.; Digumarthy, S.R.; Muse, V.V.; Kambadakone, A.R.; Blake, M.A.; Tabari, A.; Hoi, Y.; Akino, N.; Angel, E.; Madan, R.; et al. Image Quality and Lesion Detection on Deep Learning Reconstruction and Iterative Reconstruction of Submillisievert Chest and Abdominal CT. *AJR Am. J. Roentgenol.* **2020**, *214*, 566–573. [CrossRef]
8. Ludes, C.; Schaal, M.; Labani, A.; Jeung, M.Y.; Roy, C.; Ohana, M. Ultra-low dose chest CT: The end of chest radiograph? *Presse Med.* **2016**, *45*, 291–301. [CrossRef]
9. Ohana, M.; Ludes, C.; Schaal, M.; Meyer, E.; Jeung, M.Y.; Labani, A.; Roy, C. What future for chest X-ray against ultra-low-dose computed tomography? *Rev. Pneumol. Clin.* **2016**, *73*, 3–12. [CrossRef]
10. Tækker, M.; Kristjánsdóttir, B.; Graumann, O.; Laursen, C.B.; Pietersen, P.I. Diagnostic accuracy of low-dose and ultra-low-dose CT in detection of chest pathology: A systematic review. *Clin. Imaging* **2021**, *74*, 139–148. [CrossRef]
11. Lee, S.W.; Kim, Y.; Shim, S.S.; Lee, J.K.; Lee, S.J.; Ryu, Y.J.; Chang, J.H. Image quality assessment of ultra low-dose chest CT using sinogram-affirmed iterative reconstruction. *Eur. Radiol.* **2014**, *24*, 817–826. [CrossRef]
12. Messerli, M.; Kluckert, T.; Knitel, M.; Wälti, S.; Desbiolles, L.; Rengier, F.; Warschkow, R.; Bauer, R.W.; Alkadhi, H.; Leschka, S.; et al. Ultralow dose CT for pulmonary nodule detection with chest x-ray equivalent dose—A prospective intra-individual comparative study. *Eur. Radiol.* **2017**, *27*, 3290–3299. [CrossRef] [PubMed]
13. Kim, H.J.; Park, S.Y.; Lee, H.Y.; Lee, K.S.; Shin, K.E.; Moon, J.W. Ultra-Low-Dose Chest CT in Patients with Neutropenic Fever and Hematologic Malignancy: Image Quality and Its Diagnostic Performance. *Cancer Res. Treat.* **2014**, *46*, 393–402. [CrossRef] [PubMed]
14. Li, C.; Liu, B.; Meng, H.; Lv, W.; Jia, H. Efficacy and Radiation Exposure of Ultra-Low-Dose Chest CT at 100 kVp with Tin Filtration in CT-Guided Percutaneous Core Needle Biopsy for Small Pulmonary Lesions Using a Third-Generation Dual-Source CT Scanner. *J. Vasc. Interv. Radiol.* **2019**, *30*, 95–102. [CrossRef]
15. Hu-Wang, E.; Schuzer, J.L.; Rollison, S.; Leifer, E.S.; Steveson, C.; Gopalakrishnan, V.; Yao, J.; Machado, T.; Jones, A.M.; Julien-Williams, P.; et al. Chest CT Scan at Radiation Dose of a Posteroanterior and Lateral Chest Radiograph Series: A Proof of Principle in Lymphangioleiomyomatosis. *Chest* **2019**, *155*, 528–533. [CrossRef]
16. Macri, F.; Greffier, J.; Pereira, F.; Rosa, A.C.; Khasanova, E.; Claret, P.-G.; Larbi, A.; Gualdi, G.; Beregi, J.P. Value of ultra-low-dose chest CT with iterative reconstruction for selected emergency room patients with acute dyspnea. *Eur. J. Radiol.* **2016**, *85*, 1637–1644. [CrossRef] [PubMed]
17. Beregi, J.; Greffier, J. Low and ultra-low dose radiation in CT: Opportunities and limitations. *Diagn. Interv. Imaging* **2019**, *100*, 63–64. [CrossRef] [PubMed]
18. Schaal, M.; Séverac, F.; Labani, A.; Jeung, M.-Y.; Roy, C.; Ohana, M. Diagnostic Performance of Ultra-Low-Dose Computed Tomography for Detecting Asbestos-Related Pleuropulmonary Diseases: Prospective Study in a Screening Setting. *PLoS ONE* **2016**, *11*, e0168979. [CrossRef]
19. Ludes, C.; Labani, A.; Severac, F.; Jeung, M.; Leyendecker, P.; Roy, C.; Ohana, M. Ultra-low-dose unenhanced chest CT: Prospective comparison of high kV/low mA versus low kV/high mA protocols. *Diagn. Interv. Imaging* **2019**, *100*, 85–93. [CrossRef] [PubMed]
20. Meyer, E.; Labani, A.; Schaeffer, M.; Jeung, M.-Y.; Ludes, C.; Meyer, A.; Roy, C.; Leyendecker, P.; Ohana, M. Wide-volume versus helical acquisition in unenhanced chest CT: Prospective intra-patient comparison of diagnostic accuracy and radiation dose in an ultra-low-dose setting. *Eur. Radiol.* **2019**, *29*, 6858–6866. [CrossRef]
21. Martini, K.; Moon, J.; Revel, M.; Dangeard, S.; Ruan, C.; Chassagnon, G. Optimization of acquisition parameters for reduced-dose thoracic CT: A phantom study. *Diagn. Interv. Imaging* **2020**, *101*, 269–279. [CrossRef]
22. Huda, W.; Ogden, K.M.; Khorasani, M.R. Converting Dose-Length Product to Effective Dose at CT. *Radiology* **2008**, *248*, 995–1003. [CrossRef] [PubMed]
23. Hansell, D.M.; Bankier, A.A.; MacMahon, H.; McLoud, T.C.; Müller, N.L.; Remy, J. Fleischner Society: Glossary of Terms for Thoracic Imaging. *Radiology* **2008**, *246*, 697–722. [CrossRef] [PubMed]
24. Prakash, P.; Kalra, M.K.; Ackman, J.B.; Digumarthy, S.R.; Hsieh, J.; Do, S.; Shepard, J.-A.O.; Gilman, M.D. Diffuse Lung Disease: CT of the Chest with Adaptive Statistical Iterative Reconstruction Technique. *Radiology* **2010**, *256*, 261–269. [CrossRef] [PubMed]
25. Tatsugami, F.; Matsuki, M.; Nakai, G.; Inada, Y.; Kanazawa, S.; Takeda, Y.; Morita, H.; Takada, H.; Yoshikawa, S.; Fukumura, K.; et al. The effect of adaptive iterative dose reduction on image quality in 320-detector row CT coronary angiography. *Br. J. Radiol.* **2012**, *85*, e378–e382. [CrossRef] [PubMed]
26. Akagi, M.; Nakamura, Y.; Higaki, T.; Narita, K.; Honda, Y.; Awai, K. Deep learning reconstruction of equilibrium phase CT images in obese patients. *Eur. J. Radiol.* **2020**, *133*, 109349. [CrossRef] [PubMed]

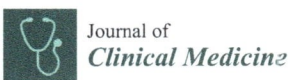

Article

Diagnostic Performance of Extracellular Volume Quantified by Dual-Layer Dual-Energy CT for Detection of Acute Myocarditis

Salim Aymeric Si-Mohamed [1,2,*], Lauria Marie Restier [3,†], Arthur Branchu [2,†], Sara Boccalini [1,2], Anaelle Congi [3], Arthur Ziegler [2], Danka Tomasevic [4], Thomas Bochaton [4], Loic Boussel [1,2] and Philippe Charles Douek [1,2]

1. Department of INSA-Lyon, University of Lyon, University Claude-Bernard Lyon 1, UJM-Saint-Étienne, CNRS, Inserm, CREATIS UMR 5220, U1206, 69621 Lyon, France; sara.boccalini@chu-lyon.fr (S.B.); loic.boussel@chu-lyon.fr (L.B.); philippe.douek@chu-lyon.fr (P.C.D.)
2. Cardiovascular and Thoracic Radiology Department, Hospices Civils de Lyon, 69500 Lyon, France; arthur.branchu@chu-lyon.fr (A.B.); arthur.ziegler69@gmail.com (A.Z.)
3. Rockfeller Faculty of Medicine, Lyon Est, University Claude-Bernard Lyon 1, 69003 Lyon, France; lauria.restier@etu.univ-lyon1.fr (L.M.R.); anaelle.congi@etu.univ-lyon1.fr (A.C.)
4. Department of Cardiology, Louis Pradel Hospital, Hospices Civils de Lyon, 59 Boulevard Pinel, 69500 Bron, France; danka.tomasevic@chu-lyon.fr (D.T.); thomas.bochaton@chu-lyon.fr (T.B.)
* Correspondence: salim.si-mohamed@chu-lyon.fr; Tel.: +33-04-7235-7335; Fax: +33-04-7235-7291
† These authors are co-second author.

Abstract: Background: Myocardial extracellular volume (ECV) is a marker of the myocarditis inflammation burden and can be used for acute myocarditis diagnosis. Dual-energy computed tomography (DECT) enables its quantification with high concordance with cardiac magnetic resonance (CMR). Purpose: To investigate the diagnostic performance of myocardial ECV quantified on a cardiac dual-layer DECT in a population of patients with suspected myocarditis, in comparison to CMR. Methods: 78 patients were included in this retrospective monocenter study, 60 were diagnosed with acute myocarditis and 18 patients were considered as a control population, based on the 2009 Lake and Louise criteria. All subjects underwent a cardiac DECT in acute phase consisted in an arterial phase followed by a late iodine enhancement phase at 10 min after injection (1.2 mL/kg, iodinated contrast agent). ECV was calculated using the hematocrit level measured the day of DECT examinations. Non-parametric analyses have been used to test the differences between groups and the correlations between the variables. A ROC curve has been used to identify the optimal ECV cut-off discriminating value allowing the detection of acute myocarditis cases. A p value < 0.05 has been considered as significant. Results: The mean ECV was significantly higher ($p < 0.001$) for the myocarditis group compared to the control (34.18 ± 0.43 vs. 30.04 ± 0.53%). A cut-off value of ECV = 31.60% (ROC AUC = 0.835, $p < 0.001$) allows to discriminate the myocarditis with a sensitivity of 80% and a specificity of 78% (positive predictive value = 92.3%, negative predictive value = 53.8% and accuracy = 79.5%). Conclusion: Myocardial ECV enabled by DECT allows to diagnose the acute myocarditis with a cut-off at 31.60% for a sensitivity of 80% and specificity of 78%.

Keywords: dual-energy CT; iodine; diagnostic imaging; myocarditis; extra-cellular volume

1. Introduction

Affecting approximately 1.8 million people worldwide in 2017 [1], myocarditis is a frequent inflammatory disease of the heart that can be caused by infectious agents, exposure to toxic substances and immune system activation [2,3]. The diagnosis includes clinical, laboratory, imaging, and histological parameters [1]; so over the years, different diagnostic tests have been developed to identify patients that have acute myocarditis. The endomyocardial biopsy has been the gold standard for a while until cardiac magnetic resonance imaging (CMR) and computed tomography (CT) got considered as non-invasive alternatives [4,5]. CMR emerged as a powerful non-invasive method for tissue characterization, including recognition and quantification of inflammation and replacement fibrosis in the setting of acute myocarditis [6,7]. Thanks to the Lake Louise Criteria, published in 2009, three markers of myocardial inflammation have been identified: hyperemia, tissue edema and necrosis/fibrosis [7]. Among the markers of the inflammatory burden, one of them stands out from the crowd: the extracellular volume (ECV).

Myocardial ECV increases related to myocardial fibroses, cardiac amyloid or edema [8]. CMR is the reference to measure ECV, but some previous studies showed that ECV can also be successfully determined with computed tomography, whether with single-energy computed tomography (SECT) or with dual-energy computed tomography (DECT), with a high correlation between ECV measurements derived from CT, histologic quantification, and CMR [9–14]. Hence, CT can effectively be considered as an interesting alternative to CMR. In addition, CT is more accessible and cheaper, while having a faster acquisition with a better spatial resolution, which makes it a good candidate for cardiac emergency imaging [15].

Therefore, we investigated the diagnostic performance of myocardial ECV quantified by cardiac DECT in a population of patients with suspected myocarditis, in comparison to CMR.

2. Materials and Methods

2.1. Study Design

This study is a monocenter retrospective study which has been conducted in the Cardiologic Hospital Louis Pradel, in Lyon (FRANCE) from May 2018 to May 2021.

2.2. Population

The population was constituted of two groups of patients that were addressed for suspicion of acute myocarditis and underwent a cardiac dual-energy computed tomography and a CMR at the acute phase: patients with confirmed acute myocarditis (MG = myocarditis group) and patients without myocarditis patterns (CG = control group). The diagnosis was confirmed according to the Lake and Louise criteria on CMR. In order to validate the diagnosis of myocarditis, the patient had to present at least two of the Lake Louise Criteria (i.e., hyperemia, tissue edema and/or fibrosis/necrosis) [7]. Exclusion criteria for the myocarditis group in order to be comparable to the control group were: an underlying cardiomyopathy and/or left ventricular ejection fraction (LVEF) ≤40% and/or acute cardiac complications (heart failure, life-threatening arrythmias, death). Exclusion criteria for the control group were: an underlying cardiomyopathy and/or LVEF <50% according to the definition of heart failure [16].

2.3. Data Registration

The following clinical, biological, functional and imaging parameters were recorded at admission: (1) age, sex, weight, size, systolic and diastolic blood pressure (SBP, DBP), heart rate, (2) values of high-sensitivity troponin (Tn), brain natriuretic peptide (BNP), creatinine; (3) left ventricular ejection fraction (LVEF) on trans-thoracic ultrasound at admission.

2.4. DECT Imaging Protocol

2.4.1. Injection Protocol

The contrast material used was Iomeprol (400 mg/mL, Iomeron®; Bracco, Milan, Italy). All patients underwent a standard coronary CT angiography injection protocol consisting on a bolus injected at 3.5 mL/s into an 18 G catheter. The injection material was followed up by a saline rinse of 20 mL. The bolus volume was calculated according to the weight of the patient (1.2 mL/kg of contrast material).

2.4.2. Image Acquisition

The examinations have been performed on a dual-layer dual-energy CT (iQon; Phillips, Haifa, Israel) consisting of a first pass arterial phase and late phase 10 min after injection. Acquisition parameters were a retrospective gated ECG acquisition at 120 kVp, with a cardiac care mas dose modulation (full dose 78%, half dose 40%), a pitch value at 0.20, and a rotation time at 0.27 s. Further technical details are provided in previous studies [17–19].

2.4.3. Reconstruction Protocol

Conventional and iodine density images were reconstructed from the late cardiac acquisition with a 1.5 mm slice thickness, a standard filter (Filter B) and a large field-of-view at 500 mm.

2.4.4. Image Analysis

Images were analyzed using a clinical workstation (Spectral Phillips Intellispace Portal Station, Phillips; Haifa, Israel). The myocardium was analyzed and manually segmented in 16 AHA segments using this software, on the iodine density images. We extracted the iodine concentrations in mg/mL for each 16 AHA segments. A circular region-of-interest of ~530 mm² was drawn in the left cardiac cavity for measuring the iodine concentration in blood. The extracellular volume (ECV) was then calculated such as following:

$$ECV = 100 \times (1 - Ht) \times \frac{\text{(Iodine concentration in the myocardium)}}{\text{(Iodine concentration in the blood)}} \quad (1)$$

The iodine concentration was measured on iodine images in mg/mL; "Ht" is the hematocrit measured the day of the DECT acquisition. From these measurements, we analyzed the global myocardial ECV-per-patient.

2.5. Radiation Dose

Dose-length-product and volume CT dose index for the late cardiac acquisition were recorded. Mean effective dose was calculated multiplying the dose-length-product by the chest k-factor of 0.014 [20].

2.6. Statistical Analyses

Statistical analyses were performed with the SPSS software (IBM SPSS Statistics 19; 2018). The data are expressed as mean ± MSE (mean standard error) and median (minimum-maximum), accordingly to the normality tests.

For comparison of continuous variables between the two study groups, a non-parametric Mann–Whitney test has been used. A non-parametric Kolmogorov–Smirnov test has been used for the nominal variables.

For correlation purposes, Spearman correlation coefficients using a 95% confidence interval were calculated between biological (BNP, creatinine), functional markers (LVEF) and the global myocardial ECV tested.

A ROC curve has been used to identify the best discriminative cut-off value of ECV and to calculate the sensitivity, the specificity, the positive predictive value, the negative predictive value and the accuracy for the diagnosis of myocarditis, after ranking all the values and linking each value to the diagnosis of myocarditis.

3. Results

3.1. Characteristics of the Population

Initially, 107 patients were addressed to the hospital for suspicion of acute myocarditis. A total 73 patients have been diagnosed with acute myocarditis while 34 patients were rules out from myocarditis on CMR. Among them, 13 patients were excluded 2 patients had a left ventricular ejection fraction ≤ 40%, 10 patients had life-threatening arrhythmia, and one patient was missing data. Finally, 60 patients have been included in the acute myocarditis group (Figure 1). Concerning the control group (CG), only 18 subjects have been included. Among the 16 patients who have not be retained for the CG, 2 of them had a left ventricular ejection fraction < 55%, 13 had cardiomyopathies and one patient had missing data (Figure 1). The baseline characteristics of the study population are summarized in Table 1.

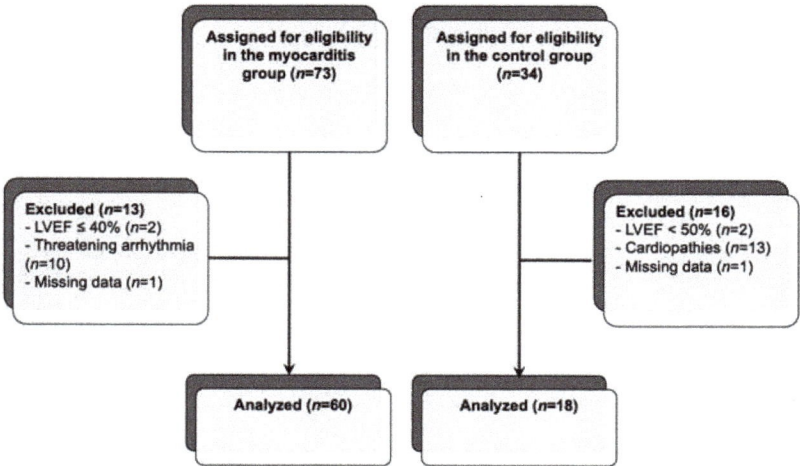

Figure 1. Flow chart of the study population.

Table 1. Baseline characteristics of the study population.

Groups		Myocarditis Group			Control Group		
Variables	n	Mean ± MSE	Median (Min–Max)	n	Mean ± MSE	Median (Min–Max)	p
Sex	60	49M, 11F		18	11M, 7F		0.602
Age (years)	60	32.9 ± 1.4	29.8 (18.0; 73.6)	18	35.1 ± 3.6	33.0 (15.0; 68.2)	0.731
Weight (kg)	60	75.0 ± 1.7	74.0 (50.0; 110.0)	18	73.8 ± 4.2	72.5 (39.0; 106.0)	0.606
Height (cm)	60	173.4 ± 1.0	173.0 (158; 194)	18	171.4 ± 2.3	172.5 (150; 185)	0.622
BMI (kg/m2)	60	24.9 ± 0.5	24.2 (17.2; 38.4)	18	24.9 ± 1.1	24.9 (17.3; 33.9)	0.962
LVEF (%)	60	57.6 ± 1.0	60.0 (42.0; 74.0)	18	64.2 ± 1.7	66.0 (55.0; 78.0)	0.006 *
Creatinine (µmol/L)	10	73.1 ± 4.1	75.0 (50.0; 88.0)	18	75.4 ± 3.8	72.0 (52.0; 111.0)	0.885
Troponins (ng/L)	60	8630.3 ± 1585.9	5365.0 (36.0; 62,929.0)	18	822.5 ± 339.9	214.5 (5.0; 5159.0)	0.001 *
BNP (ng/L)	44	137.4 ± 45.4	46.5 (0.1; 1700.0)	16	140.6 ± 76.0	35.0 (0.1; 1018.0)	0.303
Hematocrit (%)	60	42.2 ± 0.5	42.2 (33.3; 54.0)	18	42.7 ± 1.0	42.8 (35.4; 49.8)	0.589

MG = myocarditis group; CG = control group; MSE = mean standard error; BMI = body mass index; LVEF = left ventricular ejection fraction; BNP = brain natriuretic peptide; p * = significant differences (Mann–Whitney non-parametric test).

The patients of the two groups have been paired by age and sex. The mean age was 32.9 ± 1.4 years for the (MG) and respectively 35.1 ± 3.6 years for the (CG). No significant difference for mean age or male proportion has been found between the two study groups. When compared, the troponins measured level was significantly higher ($p < 0.001$; 8630.3 ± 1585.9 vs. 822.5 ± 339.9 ng/L), and the LVEF was significantly lower ($p = 0.006$; 57.6 ± 1.0 vs. 64.2 ± 1.7%) for the acute myocarditis group compared to the control group.

3.2. Measurement of the Myocardial Inflammation

Mean ECV of the myocarditis group was significantly higher compared to the one measured for the control group ($p < 0.001$, CI 95% (28.9–31.2)). Results are summarized in Table 2 and in Figure 2.

Table 2. Statistics of the ECV for both groups.

	ECV for MG ($n = 60$)	ECV for CG ($n = 18$)
Mean	34.18 *	30.04
Mean Standard Error	0.43	0.53
Median	34.61	29.93
Minimum	27.10	24.99
Maximum	40.54	33.06
25% Percentile	32.12	28.97
50% Percentile	34.61	29.93
75% Percentile	36.39	31.73

ECV = extracellular volume; MG = myocarditis group; CG = control group. Data are expressed in percentage. * Significant differences MG vs.CG (Mann–Whitney non-parametric test): $p < 0.001$.

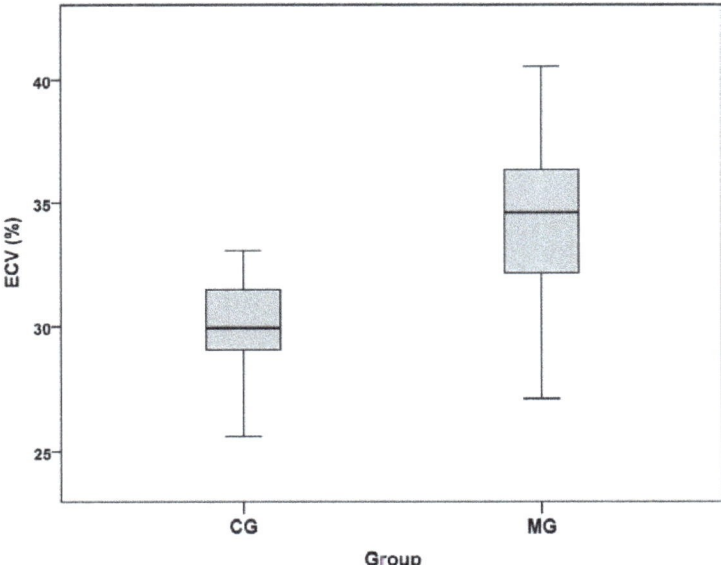

Figure 2. Box plots of the mean ECV for both groups. Median is represented by the line and the mean by the cross in the center of the box, upper and lower margins correspond to the 25th and the 75th percentiles, and outliers indicate the minimal and the maximal values. ECV = extracellular volume; CG = control group; MG = myocarditis group.

3.3. Correlation between ECV and the Different Parameters

Concerning the acute myocarditis group, a positive significant correlation ($p = 0.011$) has been found between ECV and the troponins level (Pearson coefficient = 0.325). No significant correlation between ECV and LVEF has been found for this group.

On the other hand, significant correlations (respectively $p = 0.015$ and $p = 0.048$) have been found between ECV and the weight (Pearson coefficient = -0.563) and the BMI (Pearson coefficient = -0.472). No significant correlation has been found between ECV and the troponins level for this group. All the results are summarized in Table 3.

Table 3. Spearman correlation statistics between mean ECV of each group and other parameters.

Parameters	ECV MG			ECV CG		
	n	Rho Spearman	p	n	Rho Spearman	p
Weight	60	−0.033	0.803	18	−0.423	0.080
Height	60	0.016	0.903	18	−0.362	0.140
BMI	60	−0.078	0.552	18	−0.311	0.210
Troponins	60	0.408	0.001 *	18	−0.169	0.504
LVEF	60	−0.199	0.128	18	−0.057	0.822
BNP	44	0.455	0.002 *	16	0.035	0.896

ECV = extracellular volume; MG = myocarditis group; CG = control group; n = number of observations; p = significant difference coefficient; BMI = body mass index; LVEF = left ventricular ejection fraction; BNP = brain natriuretic peptide; * = significant correlations.

3.4. Measurement of the ECV Cut-Off Value

A ROC curve has been realized to estimate the best ECV cut-off value to finally determine which value can be used to discriminate acute myocarditis in a group of patients with suspected myocarditis. This curve is significantly representative of the ECV cuts-off values ($p < 0.001$) with an area under the curve of 0.835 (with a 95% CI of (0.748–0.922)). The results are represented in the Figures 3 and 4. The retained cut-off value of 31.60% in our study has shown a sensitivity of 80%, a specificity of 78%, a positive predictive value of 92.3%, a negative predictive value of 53.8% and accuracy of 79.5% for the discrimination of acute myocarditis from the control subjects.

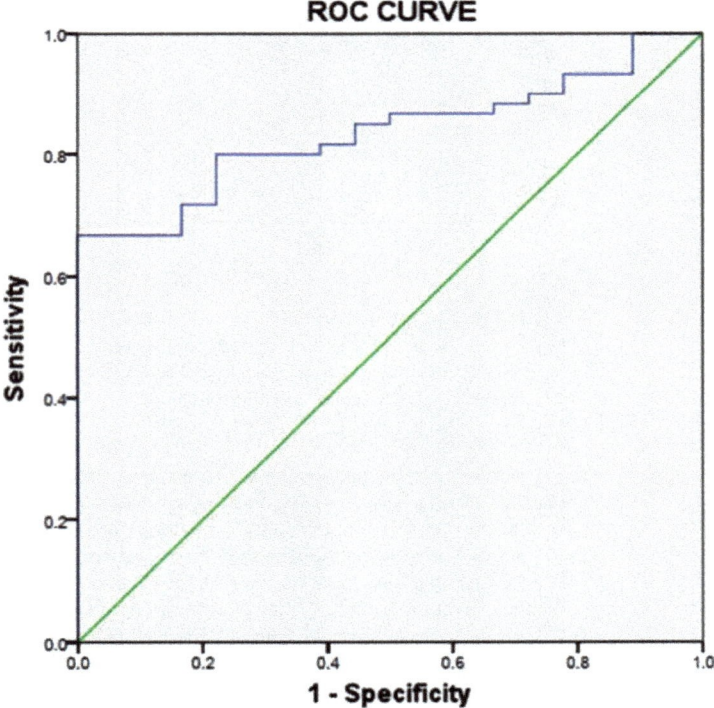

Figure 3. ROC curve representing the different cuts-off of ECV.

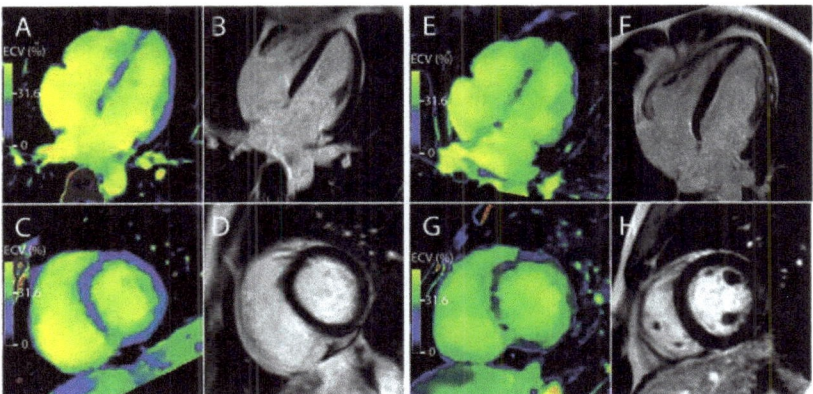

Figure 4. Representative cases of patients with suspected acute myocarditis. Left panel (**A–D**). Case of a 42-year-old woman with elevated high-sensitivity troponins at 83 ng/L at admission. A late phase DECT was performed at admission. The global ECV was measured at 29.7%. MRI did not show any late gadolinium enhancement. Right panel (**E–H**). Case of a 27-year-old man with elevated high-sensitivity troponins at 8000 ng/L at admission. A late phase DECT was performed at admission. The global ECV was measured at 35.1%. MRI showed multiple late gadolinium enhancement of the sub-epicardial myocardial wall in favor of myocarditis.

3.5. Radiation Dose Analysis

The mean ± SD volume CT dose index was 6.2 ± 1.7 mGy, the total dose length product was 123.2 ± 39.6 mGy.cm^{-1}. As a result, the mean ± SD equivalent dose was calculated to be 1.7 ± 0.5 mSv.

4. Discussion

In the present study, we showed that myocardial ECV quantified by DECT is a biomarker of the myocarditis burden and that can be used for discriminating acute myocarditis in a population of patients with suspected myocarditis. These findings support the diagnostic value of ECV in the diagnostic work-up of a suspected acute myocarditis.

The novelty of the present study is the use of CT in a suspected population of myocarditis and as so the report of ECV values which can be the starting point for its implementation in clinical routine. In the same line, few studies have reported the ECV values of different cardiopathies such as heart failure, global cardiomyopathies, cardiac amyloidosis or in aortic stenosis patients [14,21,22]. Taken together, these studies are holding great promises for cardiac CT imaging because of its many advantages. Cardiac CT allows a 3D registration along the heart muscle in a short time acquisition with an excellent spatial resolution, and direct measurement of ECV in opposition with CMR which relies on measuring the effect of GBCAs on protons [8]. Because of its poor availability and its numerous contraindications, CT seems to be an encouraging and interesting alternative to CMR despite its irradiation [23]. However, among the different CT systems, it has to be noted the great advantage for DECT technology that allows the measurement of iodine content in a tissue without requiring a pre-injection examination such as done with single-energy CT, which reduces the burden radiation dose [22,24–26]. By decomposing the X-ray spectrum in two different energies spectra, DECT systems measure the photoelectric and Compton effects. Their recombination will allow to reconstruct quantitative images of the iodine distribution in the myocardium for ECV measurement [24]. Hence, DECT imaging is more prone to cardiac tissue characterization than single-energy CT which opens the door to evaluation of the myocardial ECV.

Our results demonstrated a significant increase of ECV in acute myocarditis patients, in accordance with previous studies using CMR that underlined an elevation of this biomarker in different cardiomyopathies, including myocarditis [15,27]. We observed significant correlation between ECV and both troponins and BNP, which is coherent with the physiopathology of myocarditis. This is explained by the fact that troponins are a marker of tissue inflammation damages and BNP of a myocardial stress [7]. While for the control group, which presented a low elevation of troponins—no correlation was found. One hypothesis would be the non-flawless performances of current DECT systems for quantification of low iodine concentrations, which are reflecting low ECVs [17]. Finally, we observed a significant association between ECV and presence of myocarditis with an AUC of 83.5% ($p < 0.0001$). We have determined a cut-off value of ECV of 31.60% with high sensitivity of 80% and specificity of 78% for discriminating myocarditis. These performances are similar to different CMR studies [28–32] with pooled performances reported in a meta-analysis with a sensitivity of 76%, a specificity of 76%, a PPV of 72%, a NPV of 79% [33]. In addition, Nadjiri et al. have proposed an optimal ECV cut-off of 32.4% with a sensitivity of 93% and specificity of 74%, using CMR [28]. Altogether, the ECV values reported in the present study are in line with the data available with CMR. This is not a surprising finding, considering the high concordance between these modalities for ECV quantification as demonstrated by recent comparative studies which permits the use of this biomarker for multiple prospects [8,11,14,21]. Hence, we showed recently that ECV enabled by DECT allows a prediction of cardiac complications in acute myocarditis [34]. In this recent study, the cut-off suggested was of 39.5% which is highlighting a higher myocarditis inflammation burden that is consequently at risk. Finally, the present study is bringing one more contribution to the DECT for being a quick appropriate alternative candidate to CMR in cardiac emergency facilities [23,35].

The present study has limitations. The main limitation relies on the unperfect sensitivity of CMR using the 2009 CMR Lake Louise criteria which do not take into account ECV [7]. This limitation is mainly explained by the retrospective design of the study that started before the revised criteria in 2018 [6]. This bias probably increases ECV in the control group via false negative patients. In consequence differences between groups is probably underestimated and the bias non-differential. The absence of a fair comparison of ECV with CMR is also a limitation that points out the availability issue of CMR in acute settings reflecting a real-world practice. Yet a recent study has demonstrated similar ECV between the DECT system used in the present study and CMR, reinforcing our confidence in ECV derived from DECT scans [36]. Finally, the incremental diagnostic value of ECV by DECT to the late iodine enhancement presence has not yet been evaluated and should be performed in further studies.

As a conclusion, the evaluation of the myocardial ECV quantified by DECT in a population suspected of acute myocarditis demonstrated good diagnostic performances which allows us to consider ECV as a reliable DECT biomarker for the discrimination of myocarditis.

Author Contributions: Conceptualization, S.A.S.-M.; methodology, S.A.S.-M.; software, L.B.; validation, P.C.D., T.B.; formal analysis, A.B., A.C., S.A.S.-M., L.M.R., A.Z.; investigation, S.B., S.A.S.-M., P.C.D., L.B., D.T., A.Z.; resources, P.C.D.; data curation, P.C.D., S.A.S.-M.; writing—original draft preparation, S.A.S.-M., L.M.R., A.C., A.B.; writing—review and editing, S.A.S.-M.; supervision, S.A.S.-M., P.C.D., L.B. All authors have read and agreed to the published version of the manuscript.

Funding: This research received no external funding.

Institutional Review Board Statement: Ethical review and approval were waived for this study, due to the retrospective design of the study.

Informed Consent Statement: Written inform consent was waived by the local IRB (Hospices Civiles de Lyon) due to the retrospective design.

Conflicts of Interest: The authors declare no conflict of interest.

References

1. Golpour, A.; Patriki, D.; Hanson, P.J.; McManus, B.; Heidecker, B. Epidemiological Impact of Myocarditis. *J. Clin. Med.* **2021**, *10*, 603. [CrossRef]
2. Cooper, L.T. Myocarditis. *N. Engl. J. Med.* **2009**, *360*, 1526–1538. [CrossRef] [PubMed]
3. Caforio, A.L.P.; Pankuweit, S.; Arbustini, E.; Basso, C.; Gimeno-Blanes, J.; Felix, S.B.; Fu, M.; Heliö, T.; Heymans, S.; Jahns, R.; et al. Current state of knowledge on aetiology, diagnosis, management, and therapy of myocarditis: A position statement of the European Society of Cardiology Working Group on Myocardial and Pericardial Diseases. *Eur. Heart J.* **2013**, *34*, 2648a–2648d. [CrossRef]
4. Bozkurt, B.; Colvin, M.; Cook, J.; Cooper, L.T.; Deswal, A.; Fonarow, G.C.; Francis, G.S.; Lenihan, D.; Lewis, E.F.; McNamara, D.M.; et al. Current Diagnostic and Treatment Strategies for Specific Dilated Cardiomyopathies: A Scientific Statement From the American Heart Association. *Circulation* **2016**, *134*, e579–e646. [CrossRef]
5. Hauck, A.J.; Kearney, D.L.; Edwards, W.D. Evaluation of postmortem endomyocardial biopsy specimens from 38 patients with lymphocytic myocarditis: Implications for role of sampling error. *Mayo Clin. Proc.* **1989**, *64*, 1235–1245. [CrossRef]
6. Ferreira, V.M.; Schulz-Menger, J.; Holmvang, G.; Kramer, C.M.; Carbone I.; Sechtem, U.; Kindermann, I.; Gutberlet, M.; Cooper, L.T.; Liu, P.; et al. Cardiovascular Magnetic Resonance in Nonischemic Myocardial Inflammation: Expert Recommendations. *J. Am. Coll. Cardiol.* **2018**, *72*, 3158–3176. [CrossRef]
7. Friedrich, M.G.; Sechtem, U.; Schulz-Menger, J.; Holmvang, G.; Alakija, P.; Cooper, L.T.; White, J.A.; Abdel-Aty, H.; Gutberlet, M.; Prasad, S.; et al. Cardiovascular Magnetic Resonance in Myocarditis: A JACC White Paper. *J. Am. Coll. Cardiol.* **2009**, *53*, 1475–1487. [CrossRef]
8. Scully, P.R.; Bastarrika, G.; Moon, J.C.; Treibel, T.A. Myocardial Extracellular Volume Quantification by Cardiovascular Magnetic Resonance and Computed Tomography. *Curr. Cardiol. Rep.* **2018**, *20*, 15. [CrossRef]
9. Nacif, M.S.; Kawel, N.; Lee, J.J.; Chen, X.; Yao, J.; Zavodni, A.; Sibley, C.T.; Lima, J.A.C.; Liu, S.; Bluemke, D.A. Interstitial myocardial fibrosis assessed as extracellular volume fraction with low-radiation-dose cardiac CT. *Radiology* **2012**, *264*, 876–883. [CrossRef] [PubMed]
10. Bandula, S.; White, S.K.; Flett, A.S.; Lawrence, D.; Pugliese, F.; Ashworth, M.T.; Punwani, S.; Taylor, S.A.; Moon, J.C. Measurement of myocardial extracellular volume fraction by using equilibrium contrast-enhanced CT: Validation against histologic findings. *Radiology* **2013**, *269*, 396–403. [CrossRef]
11. Lee, H.-J.; Im, D.J.; Youn, J.-C.; Chang, S.; Suh, Y.J.; Hong, Y.J.; Kim, Y.J.; Hur, J.; Choi, B.W. Myocardial Extracellular Volume Fraction with Dual-Energy Equilibrium Contrast-enhanced Cardiac CT in Nonischemic Cardiomyopathy: A Prospective Comparison with Cardiac MR Imaging. *Radiology* **2016**, *280*, 49–57. [CrossRef]
12. Kurita, Y.; Kitagawa, K.; Kurobe, Y.; Nakamori, S.; Nakajima, H.; Dohi, K.; Ito, M.; Sakuma, H. Estimation of myocardial extracellular volume fraction with cardiac CT in subjects without clinical coronary artery disease: A feasibility study. *J. Cardiovasc. Comput. Tomogr.* **2016**, *10*, 237–241. [CrossRef]
13. Nacif, M.S.; Liu, Y.; Yao, J.; Liu, S.; Sibley, C.T.; Summers, R.M.; Bluemke, D.A. 3D left ventricular extracellular volume fraction by low-radiation dose cardiac CT: Assessment of interstitial myocardial fibrosis. *J. Cardiovasc. Comput. Tomogr.* **2013**, *7*, 51–57. [CrossRef] [PubMed]
14. Dubourg, B.; Dacher, J.-N.; Durand, E.; Caudron, J.; Bauer, F.; Bubenheim, M.; Eltchaninoff, H.; Serfaty, J.-M. Single-source dual energy CT to assess myocardial extracellular volume fraction in aortic stenosis before transcatheter aortic valve implantation (TAVI). *Diagn. Interv. Imaging* **2021**. [CrossRef] [PubMed]
15. Abadia, A.F.; van Assen, M.; Martin, S.S.; Vingiani, V.; Griffith, L.P.; Giovagnoli, D.A.; Bauer, M.J.; Schoepf, U.J. Myocardial extracellular volume fraction to differentiate healthy from cardiomyopathic myocardium using dual-source dual-energy CT. *J. Cardiovasc. Comput. Tomogr.* **2020**, *14*, 162–167. [CrossRef] [PubMed]
16. Ponikowski, P.; Voors, A.A.; Anker, S.D.; Bueno, H.; Cleland, J.G.F.; Coats, A.J.S.; Falk, V.; González-Juanatey, J.R.; Harjola, V.-P.; Jankowska, E.A.; et al. 2016 ESC Guidelines for the diagnosis and treatment of acute and chronic heart failure: The Task Force for the diagnosis and treatment of acute and chronic heart failure of the European Society of Cardiology (ESC)Developed with the special contribution of the Heart Failure Association (HFA) of the ESC. *Eur. Heart J.* **2016**, *37*, 2129–2200. [CrossRef]
17. Si-Mohamed, S.; Dupuis, N.; Tatard-Leitman, V.; Rotzinger, D.; Boccalini, S.; Dion, M.; Vlassenbroek, A.; Coulon, P.; Yagil, Y.; Shapira, N.; et al. Virtual versus true non-contrast dual-energy CT imaging for the diagnosis of aortic intramural hematoma. *Eur. Radiol.* **2019**. [CrossRef]
18. Rotzinger, D.C.; Si-Mohamed, S.A.; Shapira, N.; Douek, P.C.; Meuli, R.A.; Boussel, L. "Dark-blood" dual-energy computed tomography angiography for thoracic aortic wall imaging. *Eur. Radiol.* **2020**, *30*, 425–431. [CrossRef] [PubMed]
19. Rotzinger, D.C.; Si-Mohamed, S.A.; Yerly, J.; Boccalini, S.; Becce, F.; Boussel, L.; Meuli, R.A.; Qanadli, S.D.; Douek, P.C. Reduced-iodine-dose dual-energy coronary CT angiography: Qualitative and quantitative comparison between virtual monochromatic and polychromatic CT images. *Eur. Radiol.* **2021**. [CrossRef]
20. Bongartz, G.; Golding, S.J.; Jurik, A.G.; Leonardi, M.; van Meerten, E.v.P. European Guidelines on Quality Criteria for Computed Tomography. Available online: http://www.drs.dk/guidelines/ct/quality/htmlindex.htm (accessed on 26 March 2020).
21. Wang, R.; Liu, X.; Schoepf, U.J.; van Assen, M.; Alimohamed, I.; Griffith, L.P.; Luo, T.; Sun, Z.; Fan, Z.; Xu, L. Extracellular volume quantitation using dual-energy CT in patients with heart failure: Comparison with 3T cardiac MR. *Int. J. Cardiol.* **2018**, *268*, 236–240. [CrossRef]

22. Scully, P.R.; Patel, K.P.; Saberwal, B.; Klotz, E.; Augusto, J.B.; Thornton, G.D.; Hughes, R.K.; Manisty, C.; Lloyd, G.; Newton, J.D.; et al. Identifying Cardiac Amyloid in Aortic Stenosis. *JACC Cardiovasc. Imaging* **2020**, *13*, 2177–2189. [CrossRef]
23. Esposito, A.; Palmisano, A.; Barbera, M.; Vignale, D.; Benedetti, G.; Spoladore, R.; Ancona, M.B.; Giannini, F.; Oppizzi, M.; Del Maschio, A.; et al. Cardiac Computed Tomography in Troponin-Positive Chest Pain: Sometimes the Answer Lies in the Late Iodine Enhancement or Extracellular Volume Fraction Map. *JACC. Cardiovasc. Imaging* **2019**, *12*, 745–748. [CrossRef] [PubMed]
24. Si-Mohamed, S.A.; Douek, P.C.; Boussel, L. Spectral CT: Dual energy CT towards multienergy CT. *J. Imag. Diagn. Interv.* **2019**, *2*, 32–45. [CrossRef]
25. Si-Mohamed, S.; Bar-Ness, D.; Sigovan, M.; Cormode, D.P.; Coulon, P.; Coche, E.; Vlassenbroek, A.; Normand, G.; Boussel, L.; Douek, P. Review of an initial experience with an experimental spectral photon-counting computed tomography system. *Nucl. Instrum. Methods Phys. Res. Sect. A Accel. Spectrometers Detect. Assoc. Equip.* **2017**, *873*, 27–35. [CrossRef]
26. Si-Mohamed, S.; Moreau-Triby, C.; Tylski, P.; Tatard-Leitman, V.; Wdowik, Q.; Boccalini, S.; Dessouky, R.; Douek, P.; Boussel, L. Head-to-head comparison of lung perfusion with dual-energy CT and SPECT-CT. *Diagn. Interv. Imaging* **2020**, *101*, 299–310. [CrossRef]
27. Gräni, C.; Bière, L.; Eichhorn, C.; Kaneko, K.; Agarwal, V.; Aghayev, A.; Steigner, M.; Blankstein, R.; Jerosch-Herold, M.; Kwong, R.Y. Incremental value of extracellular volume assessment by cardiovascular magnetic resonance imaging in risk stratifying patients with suspected myocarditis. *Int. J. Cardiovasc. Imaging* **2019**, *35*, 1067–1078. [CrossRef] [PubMed]
28. Nadjiri, J.; Nieberler, H.; Hendrich, E.; Greiser, A.; Will, A.; Martinoff, S.; Hadamitzky, M. Performance of native and contrast-enhanced T1 mapping to detect myocardial damage in patients with suspected myocarditis: A head-to-head comparison of different cardiovascular magnetic resonance techniques. *Int. J. Cardiovasc. Imaging* **2017**, *33*, 539–547. [CrossRef] [PubMed]
29. Luetkens, J.A.; Doerner, J.; Thomas, D.K.; Dabir, D.; Gieseke, J.; Sprinkart, A.M.; Fimmers, R.; Stehning, C.; Homsi, R.; Schwab, J.O.; et al. Acute myocarditis: Multiparametric cardiac MR imaging. *Radiology* **2014**, *273*, 383–392. [CrossRef]
30. Radunski, U.K.; Lund, G.K.; Stehning, C.; Schnackenburg, B.; Bohnen, S.; Adam, G.; Blankenberg, S.; Muellerleile, K. CMR in patients with severe myocarditis: Diagnostic value of quantitative tissue markers including extracellular volume imaging. *JACC Cardiovasc. Imaging* **2014**, *7*, 667–675. [CrossRef]
31. Lurz, P.; Luecke, C.; Eitel, I.; Föhrenbach, F.; Frank, C.; Grothoff, M.; de Waha, S.; Rommel, K.-P.; Lurz, J.A.; Klingel, K.; et al. Comprehensive Cardiac Magnetic Resonance Imaging in Patients With Suspected Myocarditis: The MyoRacer-Trial. *J. Am. Coll. Cardiol.* **2016**, *67*, 1800–1811. [CrossRef]
32. von Knobelsdorff-Brenkenhoff, F.; Schüler, J.; Dogangüzel, S.; Dieringer, M.A.; Rudolph, A.; Greiser, A.; Kellman, P.; Schulz-Menger, J. Detection and Monitoring of Acute Myocarditis Applying Quantitative Cardiovascular Magnetic Resonance. *Circ. Cardiovasc. Imaging* **2017**, *10*, e005242. [CrossRef] [PubMed]
33. Pan, J.A.; Lee, Y.J.; Salerno, M. Diagnostic Performance of Extracellular Volume, Native T1, and T2 Mapping versus Lake Louise Criteria by CMR for Detection of Acute Myocarditis: A Meta-Analysis. *Circ. Cardiovasc. Imaging* **2018**, *11*, e007598. [CrossRef] [PubMed]
34. Si-Mohamed, S.A.; Congi, A.; Ziegler, A.; Tomasevic, D.; Tatard-Leitman, V.; Broussaud, T.; Boccalini, S.; Bensalah, M.; Rouvière, A.-S.; Bonnefoy-Cudraz, E.; et al. Early Prediction of Cardiac Complications in Acute Myocarditis by Means of Extracellular Volume Quantification With the Use of Dual-Energy Computed Tomography. *JACC Cardiovasc. Imaging* **2021**. [CrossRef]
35. Bouleti, C.; Baudry, G.; Iung, B.; Arangalage, D.; Abtan, J.; Ducrocq, G.; Steg, P.-G.; Vahanian, A.; Henry-Feugeas, M.-C.; Pasi, N.; et al. Usefulness of Late Iodine Enhancement on Spectral CT in Acute Myocarditis. *JACC Cardiovasc. Imaging* **2017**, *10*, 826–827. [CrossRef] [PubMed]
36. Oda, S.; Emoto, T.; Nakaura, T.; Kidoh, M.; Utsunomiya, D.; Funama, Y.; Nagayama, Y.; Takashio, S.; Ueda, M.; Yamashita, T.; et al. Myocardial Late Iodine Enhancement and Extracellular Volume Quantification with Dual-Layer Spectral Detector Dual-Energy Cardiac CT. *Radiol. Cardiothorac. Imaging* **2019**, *1*, e180003. [CrossRef] [PubMed]

MDPI
St. Alban-Anlage 66
4052 Basel
Switzerland
Tel. +41 61 683 77 34
Fax +41 61 302 89 18
www.mdpi.com

Journal of Clinical Medicine Editorial Office
E-mail: jcm@mdpi.com
www.mdpi.com/journal/jcm

www.ingramcontent.com/pod-product-compliance
Lightning Source LLC
LaVergne TN
LVHW070554100526
838202LV00012B/467